The Psychiatric
Mental Status
Examination

The Psychiatric Mental Status Examination

Paula T. Trzepacz, M.D.
Robert W. Baker, M.D.

New York   Oxford
OXFORD UNIVERSITY PRESS
1993

Oxford University Press

Oxford   New York   Toronto
Delhi   Bombay   Calcutta   Madras   Karachi
Kuala Lumpur   Singapore   Hong Kong   Tokyo
Nairobi   Dar es Salaam   Cape Town
Melbourne   Auckland   Madrid

and associated companies in
Berlin   Ibadan

Trzepacz, Paula T.
Psychiatric mental status examination / Paula T. Trzepacz, Robert W. Baker.
p.   cm.   Includes bibliographical references and index
ISBN 0-19-506251-5
1. Mental illness—Diagnosis.   2. Interviewing in psychiatry.
3. Psychodiagnostics.   I. Baker, Robert W., 1958- .   II. Title.
[DNLM: 1. Interview, Psychological—methods.   2. Mental Disorders—
diagnosis.   WM 141 T876p]
RC469.T79   1993
616.89075—dc20
DNLM/DLC
for Library of Congress   92-48947

9 8 7 6 5 4 3

Printed in the United States of America
on acid-free paper

This book was written in honor of our parents, Mary P. Trzepacz and the late Edward J. Trzepacz, and Martha C. Baker and Robert J. Baker, M.D.

We dedicate this book to our patients, whom we hope will benefit from the ever-increasing knowledge about psychiatric disorders and their treatment, and for whom we hope the stigma of having mental illness will forever diminish.

Preface

This text has grown from years of teaching psychiatry to medical students and residents. Learning to perform a mental status examination is an important prerequisite to clinical work, analogous to the physical examination. Though it is covered briefly in psychiatric texts, we believe that a current and thorough text devoted solely to describing components of the psychiatric mental status examination (MSE) is sorely needed. Previously published books focusing on MSE issues include texts with a psychoanalytic approach, a programed self-teaching guide that does not follow the traditional format, and texts that integrate some mental status information with interviewing techniques and differential diagnosis. This comprehensive text on the MSE should fill a void in the teaching literature and be useful to both students first learning about the MSE, and seasoned clinicians seeking an advanced reference.

The psychiatric MSE is actually a section of a comprehensive medical examination, though in this context it often receives cursory, if any, attention. In order to complete an adequate MSE, one must have knowledge of psychiatric terminology and phenomenology, be able to detect or elicit necessary data during the assessment interview, and know how to interpret and integrate these data in a clinically meaningful way. In addition to completing and understanding the MSE, students of psychiatric medicine should learn to describe their findings in a predictable, concise, and unambiguous manner. The vocabulary and organization used in MSE reports may vary slightly from one physician to another, but overall are quite similar.

Appropriate vocabulary and organization are described in this text. We have strived to be as accurate and up-to-date as possible, but it is important to realize that a given term or concept may be understood differently in different settings, and two or more terms may have similar or overlapping meanings: For example, terms preferred by psychiatrists may overlap but are not necessarily congruent with terms used by neurologists. Particular care should be exercised when interpreting our comments about diagnosis and management, as they are not the central focus of our book and are mentioned only as examples to put MSE data into a clinical context. Diagnostic and treatment decisions should be made upon consideration of the whole clinical picture and be based on the physician's training and experience and, when necessary, supervision.

This book is meant to be practical and "user friendly" in its approach. After an introductory chapter, this text is divided into six chapters that focus separately on the sections of the MSE. Each chapter, representing a section of the MSE, provides examples of psychiatric conditions with their described signs and symptoms. Detailed definitions of important terminology are listed at the end of each chapter. These definitions provide the vocabulary necessary to communicate findings briefly and clearly to other physicians. The final chapter describes hypothetical case vignettes and sample MSEs to illustrate how all this information is written into a medical record. The Appendix outlines the process of information-gathering and recording of the MSE during actual patient care.

An important feature of this book is the conclusion of each chapter, which provides definitions specifically relevant to that section of the MSE. Students may wish to skim them *before* reading each chapter and refer to them again as needed while reading the chapter. Advanced practitioners can use these definitions as a reference. These definitions are generally more comprehensive and integrative than those found in a dictionary. Because they are topically organized, and thus grouped according to clinical relevance, they act as a study guide for the beginning student.

The organization of the MSE enables the psychiatrist to describe objectively what has been seen and heard during the patient interview. Although this text includes some sample questions for eliciting information, it is not intended to instruct the reader in interview techniques. Interviewing is a necessary skill, but it is a large topic that is covered more thoroughly in other texts devoted specifically to that topic. Some of these are cited in the references for Chapter 1.

This book may be useful for medical students, residents, and practicing physicians (in the fields of psychiatry, neurology, internal medicine, and family practice), as well as for psychologists, social workers, psychiatric nurses, and others who come into contact with patients.

We would like to thank our colleagues for taking the time to preview and critique our work: James Baird, Ph.D., for his suggestions on the Cognition chapter; Roy Chengappa, M.D., for his comments on the Thought Content and Process chapter; Cyndie Spanier, M.S., for her comments on the Speech and Language chapter; and Robert J. Baker, M.D., for his comments on the Insight and Judgment chapter. Finally, we could not have accomplished the writing of this book without the advice of, encouragement from, and editing by our delightful and patient editor, Joan Bossert.

Pittsburgh, Pa.   P.T.T.
September 1992   R.W.B.

Contents

The Psychiatric Mental Status Examination

1 | What Is a Mental Status Examination?

Learning the Mental Status Examination

The beginning student of the mental status examination (MSE) faces a task like that of an aspiring music critic. Anyone can listen to and even enjoy a symphony orchestra. However, professionally reviewing its performance takes special knowledge, vocabulary, and skills. The critic requires both textbook facts (e.g., Which instruments are which? Who are the Baroque composers?) and an adequate vocabulary to describe unambiguously musical or technical observations. In addition, skilled music critics have learned a higher level of auditory observation: attending to nuances of individual notes while placing them in the context of melodies and harmonies; recognizing and analyzing the product of individual instruments while simultaneously considering the interplay of the entire orchestra; and understanding the piece's structure and themes. Similarly, anyone can have a conversation with a patient, but appropriate knowledge, vocabulary, and skills can elevate the clinician's "conversation" to a "mental status examination."

This textbook provides the basic knowledge and vocabulary that students require to organize and describe an MSE; it also provides some guideposts to the performance of the examination. This book should serve as a starting point and reference point for the MSE; however, skillful performance of the examination is honed with practice, experience, and supervision.

Like attentive listeners to symphonic music, experienced clinicians attend to detail and subtlety in behavior, such as the affect accompanying thoughts or ideas, the significance of gesture or mannerism, and the unspoken message of conversation. The MSE allows the organization, completion, and communication of these observations.

The Mental Status Examination

Successful evaluation and treatment of psychopathologic symptoms, cognitive impairment, and emotional distress can be based only on thorough and objective assessment of the patient, utilizing the MSE. Unfortunately, physicians who are challenged by psychiatric patients may feel better prepared to deal with somatic symptoms than with psychiatric ones.

A medical or psychiatric history and physical examination aim to elucidate signs and symptoms. A *sign* is an objective finding with specific connotations; for

Table 1.1. Sections of a written psychiatric evaluation

Subjective:	Chief complaint
	History of present illness
	Past medical and psychiatric history
	Social history
	Family history
	Review of systems
Objective:	Physical examination
	Mental status examination
	Laboratory tests
	Radiologic and other tests
Assessment:	Discussion of case
	Differential diagnosis
Plan:	Further assessment
	Testing
	Treatments

example, the extensor plantar reflex is indicative of an upper motor neuron lesion. Similarly, loose associations are a sign of thought disorder, and an inability to recall three objects after a few minutes is a sign of memory disturbance. The term *symptom* is broader than sign. Some regard symptoms as complaints and other significant subjective reports offered by the patient, as opposed to objective findings of an examination by a physician. However, in common usage, the term "symptom" refers to any datum suggestive of the presence of disease and, thus, includes signs as well as reports by the patient.

Psychiatric signs and symptoms are not necessarily mysterious or daunting, especially if approached systematically. Table 1–1 suggests an outline for organizing psychiatric evaluations. This is quite similar to the standard outline for medical evaluations. The role of the MSE in the investigation of psychiatric problems is analogous to that played by the physical examination in the investigation of somatic problems.

The psychiatric MSE is the component of the psychiatric evaluation that includes observing the patient's behavior and describing it in an objective, non-judgmental manner. Like the physical examination, the MSE seeks to reveal signs of illness. Like the physical examination, the MSE is termed the *objective* portion of the patient evaluation, even though the elicited data vary with the clinician's ability, style, and training. In contrast, the *case history* is the *subjective* portion of the psychiatric evaluation, based on the patient's experiences and memory (*anamnesis*) of them. This information is considered subjective because in relating it, patients are biased by their understanding, experiences, intellect, and personality. The history includes patients' psychiatric problems as presented at the time of the examination; current functioning; ongoing medical problems and medications; past medical, surgical, obstetric, and psychiatric information;

social history; family history; a review of organ systems; and a review of major categories of potential psychiatric symptoms.

Unlike the physical examination, the MSE is not conducted as a completely separate portion of the patient evaluation. Much of the information needed for a MSE is gathered during the course of the interview, and the performance of the examination is integrated into the whole interview process. Some of the MSE is completed simply through observation of the patient—for example, noting the manner of dress or facial expression. Other aspects of the examination require specific testing or questioning. For example, portions of the speech and language and the cognitive examinations are often performed separately because specific tests of language, attention, memory, calculations, and so on, are needed. History from the patient, family, caregivers, previous doctors and therapists, and medical records can alert the psychiatrist to areas of pathology that need further exploration. Yet, unlike the history, which includes past as well as current information, the MSE is an evaluation of the *current* state of the patient, which consists of observations made during that evaluation session.

Usefulness of the Mental Status Examination

The information gathered from an MSE is used in conjunction with other objective data, such as findings from the physical examination, laboratory tests, neuropsychologic testing, electrophysiological testing, and radiologic and nuclear medicine testing. Only by combining subjective and objective data is an adequate knowledge base assembled to permit diagnosis of the disorders or conditions that may be affecting the patient. Once a differential diagnosis is established, further testing can be ordered as needed and appropriate treatment begun. (Because this book is not intended as a treatise on psychiatric differential diagnosis, the reader is referred to psychiatric texts and to the American Psychiatric Association's (1987) publication *Diagnostic and Statistical Manual, Third Edition, Revised* which is also known as *DSM-III-R*. *DSM-III-R* describes the inclusion and exclusion criteria for psychiatric diagnoses. The next edition, *DSM-IV*, is in preparation.)

A complete and thorough MSE is necessary for evaluating emotional, behavioral, or cognitive disorders, but any careful medical evaluation should include elements of the MSE. It is perhaps a physician's best tool for uncovering inapparent neuropsychiatric impairment. Whether because of training or disposition, many physicians unfortunately find themselves more at ease in conducting a physical examination than an MSE. The latter is frequently recorded in the chart as "alert and oriented times three,"* omitting many areas that require screening (e.g., disturbance of mood or attention).

*"Oriented times three" is a conventional synonym for fully oriented; it alludes to three general areas of orientation: person, place, and time. Orientation is discussed in Chapter 6.

Not only does the MSE often provide information critical for making a differential diagnosis, but also, once a baseline MSE is done, serial performance of the examination over time permits an objective reassessment of the patient's condition and response to treatment. Changes in the MSE findings should reflect changes in the patient's condition.

Conducting the MSE may also clarify the reliability of the historical information being gathered during the interview itself. For example, a mildly demented patient may give inaccurate information that, if taken at face value, would mislead the interviewer. Memory problems might preclude accurate historical reporting by such a patient, but may not be apparent unless the examiner utilizes a cognitive/behavioral assessment, as formalized in an MSE. When working with any patient in whom it is suspected that dementia may be interfering with the validity of the history, the examiner should proceed immediately to the cognitive examination portion of the MSE (see Chapter 6). Family members, neighbors, caregivers, and doctors may then need to be contacted to obtain accurate historical information.

The Interview as a Means to Elicit Information

The psychiatric MSE entails a clinical rather than social approach to the patient. The examiner closely listens to what is said and not said, structuring the examination in a way that allows broad exploration in many areas for potential abnormalities, as well as in-depth exploration of evident symptoms or signs. The patient is critically observed; behaviors that are either ignored out of politeness or simply not noticed in social situations must be carefully attended to and described during the psychiatric MSE. On the other hand, in reporting the MSE, global statements that might be made in social contexts (e.g., "he's weird") are inadequate and judgmental in the clinical setting.

The interviewer's technique is important in eliciting information during the MSE. While a thorough review of interview technique is beyond the scope of this book (see suggested references at end of chapter), some general comments can be made. Most important, the interviewer should strive to form a therapeutic alliance so that patients can feel reasonably comfortable expressing themselves and sharing personal information. Generally psychiatrists prefer to allow patients unstructured time at the beginning of the interview to explain what is bothering them. This can be accomplished by asking open-ended questions such as, "Tell me how you have been feeling since your wife died?" After a few minutes, the interviewer can ask specific questions to guide the patient into relevant areas of inquiry; for example, "How many pills did you take in a day?" or "How has your mood been recently?" Some patients may need to be encouraged or gently prodded into discussing certain topics, such as sexual matters, violent thoughts, or suicidal ideation. Empathic comments interspersed throughout the interview will reveal to patients that the interviewer can understand what they have been going through, and that the interviewer is interested in what they are saying. Empathic comments—"It sounds as though you felt very discouraged; did you feel like life wasn't worth living anymore?"—also encourage the patient to continue talking about a difficult topic. In fact, performance of an MSE often communicates the examiner's interest in the patient, and signals authorization to discuss emotional issues.

Certain topics such as suicidality, homocidality, "crazy" thoughts or ideas, and intimate details of interpersonal relationships may be avoided by the interviewer out of hesitancy or awkwardness. It is important not to miss such vital information. As the interview is not a social occasion, it is not governed by social norms of politeness. The interviewer should attempt to display calm, comfort, and objectivity when these questions are posed, in order to communicate to patients that all aspects of their lives are relevant. Patients may collude with an uncomfortable interviewer in avoiding sensitive topics; consequent withholding of feelings such as suicidality could be dangerous. Suicidal patients commonly feel relieved by the physician's inquiry about suicidality, as it offers a welcome opportunity to discuss these feelings.

The interviewer should assure the patient that disclosures are confidential, to the extent that the circumstance allow. Certainly, threatened harm to self or others requires balancing the need for confidentiality against the need to inform other persons, such as family, friends, police, or the intended victim. These contingencies usually should be made known to the patient. It is often useful to inform the patient that under certain conditions confidentiality will need to be broken; generally, a threat of harm to self or others is a reason to protect the patient from acting on such feelings.

Different types of patients require different styles of interviewing. Paranoid patients may be suspicious, frightened, and distrusting. They will need to be reassured that they are safe, and that they will not be trapped in the room by the examiner; with such patients, it is prudent to maintain more physical distance and less continuous eye contact than usual. Demented patients may not completely comprehend the questions asked; they may become hostile as a defense against revealing the inadequacy of their cognitive abilities. Depressed patients tend to view the world through gray-colored glasses, have decreased interest and motivation, and have poor judgment about their own welfare; because they may care little about life, they are often poorly motivated in responding to questions; if they fail spontaneously to discuss themselves, probing questions are required. Manic patients may be irritable, sarcastic, inappropriately jocular, and psychomotorically agitated, making it difficult to engage their cooperation.

While much of the MSE information can be elicited by direct questioning of the patient, some must be inferred from context and from the patient's behavior. For example, a delirious patient may be too frightened or confused to describe visual hallucinations; yet the trained observer will suspect them if the patient keeps suddenly looking away, apparently attending to a stimulus not observable to others. At other times it may be necessary to "read between the lines" by thinking about the implications of verbal statements; for example, the examiner may detect paranoid thinking to which the patient alludes but will not directly admit.

The skillful examiner will attend to both the content and the process of the interview. *Content* is the overtly communicated information, while *process* is how the communications occur. Process includes feelings, innuendos, and behaviors that accompany speech and thought. For every thought there is an accompanying feeling; thoughts form the content, while emotions contribute to the process. Feelings may not be verbalized and may instead be expressed by actions. In addition, the content and process may not always be congruent. For example, a patient may deny feeling depressed while looking sad and crying. Another patient may smile and state that his or her marriage is a happy one, while glaring at the physician and using a hostile tone of voice because he or she was questioned about this sensitive topic. In each of these cases, the stated message or content does not match the process, and the psychiatrist should record this observation of incongruency in addition to what the patient overtly admits. There are useful data generated by listening to both the overt verbalized information (content) and also to indirect information expressed (process). Careful observation of nonverbal behavior and reading between the lines are required to detect the process. Often the process is more accurate than the content in reflecting what the patient really thinks and feels.

It is also useful for physicians to monitor objectively their own feelings and reactions during the interview. An examiner's "gut reactions" may signal subtle emotions being expressed by the patient. For example, a depressed patient often makes the examiner feel sad. An angry and hostile patient may behave in a manner that makes the examiner feel threatened and angry, whereas a manipulative patient may make the examiner feel perturbed, irritated, or coerced. These evoked feelings are part of the useful information to be assimilated during the assessment. Although the physician needs to be aware of such feelings, it is very important to be cautious not to react countertherapeutically toward the patient because of these evoked feelings. This would be "acting out" one's own feelings—an inappropriate, unprofessional response.

The Clinician's Demeanor

Traditional psychoanalytic practice requires the analyst to behave in a distant, unemotional, and quiet manner, giving very little information or very few responses to the patient; this approach has been called the "blank slate." This style is unfortunately what many expect from psychiatrists, since it has been popularized by the media. This is not the predominant style in modern psychiatric practice. In fact, psychoanalysis is a specific technique reserved only for a minority of relatively intact patients who can withstand the distance and anonymity of the analyst as they explore their own personalities and past experiences. Most psychiatrists are not analysts (this requires special training).

We do not advocate an analytic approach to interviewing patients. Instead, it is expected that the physician performing an MSE interview is an active participant. It is true that, in general, psychiatrists should not talk about themselves, their own experiences, or their personal opinions with patients. To this extent the psychiatrist remains anonymous to the patient, and the information given by the patient is untainted by knowledge about the physician. Yet, the individual therapeutic style should remain flexible according to the clinical situation. For example, a paranoid, psychotic patient seen in an emergency room setting would be handled with therapeutic distance and without familiarity, which might overwhelm the patient. On the other hand, a depressed patient in the general hospital who is dying from cancer could be approached with warmth, openness, and even a touch to the hand during particularly sad moments.

The physician should attempt to remain calm through the interview, regardless of whether the patient is angry, irritable, agitated, hostile, anxious, or euphoric. Comments that placidly reflect back to the patient what is observed about the patient's feelings are appropriate. This should be done in an objective and nonthreatening manner; for example: "You are obviously quite upset about this," or "Do you feel safe here?" Calmness in the face of turmoil also signals that the examiner is in control, even if the patient is not.

The examiner should behave professionally and avoid behaving in a judgmental manner during the interview, trying not to be caught off guard when something unexpectedly funny occurs. Occasionally, a psychotic or manic patient will say something that is comical, and it is difficult not to smile or laugh. In such an instance, one would hopefully be laughing at the comment and not at the patient.

More on Interviewing Patients

The MSE should quickly screen many areas of possible abnormality as well as closely investigate those areas of probable abnormality. Good examiners think about likely differential diagnoses from their very first contact with the patient; their examinations are broad enough to screen all areas, but focus on questions and observations that help exclude or verify potential conclusions. This can be likened to the physical examination of a patient with a breathing difficulty; a careful and discriminating approach should be taken to the oropharyngeal, cardiovascular, and respiratory systems, but the remaining examination, such as investigation of the abdomen and reflexes, should not be entirely neglected. As a consequence, the MSE is not a preprogramed procedure, but a variable and dynamic entity that is shaped by the physician's interpersonal relationship with the patient and guided by his or her diagnostic hypotheses.

Experienced interviewers usually follow their patients' leads, matching their questions more or less logically to the preceding dialogue. Patients may be quickly alienated by physicians who appear to conform to their own script rather than seeming interested and inquisitive about the patient's concerns. It is generally appropriate to be open-ended in questions at the start of an interview, and to attempt to follow up on statements that seem important to the patient. On the other hand, keeping the overall structure of the MSE in mind can help ensure a comprehensive screening.

The MSE, along with relevant information from history and physical and ancillary or laboratory examinations, provides the foundation for diagnostic and prognostic decisions. The examiner should be consciously aware of diagnostic, treatment, and safety considerations that help in framing questions. Beyond basic screening, questions should refute or confirm hypotheses generated in the course of the examination. For example, if an elderly depressed patient reports improved mood and sleep but new absentmindedness and distractibility since starting a tricyclic antidepressant, it would be important to test the hypothesis that the new complaints reflect anticholinergic toxicity. This could be done by carefully evaluating attention and memory, as well as pursuing relevant history and physical findings, such as dry mouth, mydriasis, or tachycardia. Similarly, in the paranoid patient who describes persecution by others, one should focus on potential dangerousness, such as by asking about steps that the patient has taken to protect himself or about urges he has had to kill his supposed persecutors.

The Written Mental Status Examination

When documenting the psychiatric evaluation in the patient's medical record, the organizational format listed in Table 1–1 is recommended. The MSE should immediately follow the physical examination and should be written in a professional and objective manner using terminology that is nonprejudicial, and nonjudgmental of the patient in a moral or ethical sense. Examples of appropriate wording will be given throughout this book.

It is important, too, that the MSE be recorded in a structured fashion and divided into discrete sections (see Table 1–2). Use of a structured format, such as the conventional format described in this book, helps the psychiatrist avoid oversights and makes the MSE readable and organized for others involved in treating the patient. Desired information can then be found quickly, in an expected location. Specific, conventional terminology will help in communicating to others just what is meant by the examiner who records the MSE. In this way, the information is standardized. The use of such terms also helps to avoid

Table 1.2. Sections of the mental status examination

Appearance, Attitude, and Activity
Mood and Affect
Speech and Language
Thought Process, Thought Content, and Perception
Cognition
Insight and Judgment

the pitfall of potential bias toward the patient evident in some judgmental descriptors.

The written MSE becomes part of a medicolegal document that can be read in court or by the patient. More important, it constitutes a communication of the patient's mental state for other physicians and caregivers.

Organization of This Text

Although the MSE is not standardized, this text describes the conventional parts of an MSE as practiced by a majority of psychiatrists. Most learn how to perform an MSE during medical school and residency training by observing others and through lectures. This book will help to teach the art of doing an MSE and offer some sense of standardization to those who are learning about it for the first time. In addition, at the end of each chapter, it offers readers detailed definitions of the vocabulary that can be used to describe the MSE. Examples of various disorders that are associated with different signs and symptoms are presented throughout the text. In this way, practitioners can become conversant with the descriptors used by psychiatric physicians performing an MSE. Chapter 8 includes case vignettes and sample MSEs so that the reader can learn how to apply information gleaned from a clinical context to a simulated MSE written into a medical record.

The portions of the MSE can be divided into the following sections: Appearance, Attitude, and Activity; Mood and Affect; Speech and Language; Thought Process, Thought Content, and Perception; Cognition; and Insight and Judgment. In this book, a separate chapter will be devoted to each of these of these sections of the MSE. Some topics would seem to fit into more than one chapter. The decision to include certain information in one chapter instead of another is usually based on tradition. For example, suicidal ideation is discussed under thought content, but is also logically related to mood and affect. Similarly, hallucinations are considered part of thought content and process, though others might choose to include them under cognition or in a separate chapter on perception. Because of such overlap, there is some variation in MSE organization from region to region and even physician to physician. Nevertheless, it is invaluable for the student to adopt, memorize, and practice a structured organization for the MSE such as that suggested here. Such a structure lends order and predictability to a potentially chaotic and daunting task.

This text can provide the vocabulary, organization, and method necessary for a good MSE; to perform the examination competently, the clinician should supplement this information with practice, supervision, and the study of psychiatric disorders.

References

American Psychiatric Association. *Diagnostic and Statistical Manual of Mental Disorders* (Third Edition-Revised), DSM-III-R. Washington, D.C.: American Psychiatric Press, 1987.

Campbell, R. J. *Psychiatry Dictionary*, 6th edition. New York: Oxford University Press, 1989.

Enelow, A. J., and Swisher, S. N. *Interviewing and Patient Care*, 3rd edition. New York: Oxford University Press, 1986.

MacKinnon, R. A., and Michels R. *The Psychiatric Interview in Clinical Practice*. Philadelphia: W. B. Saunders, 1971.

Othmer, E., and Othmer, S. C. *The Clinical Interview Using DSM-III-R*. Washington, D.C.: American Psychiatric Press, 1989.

Shea, S. C. *Psychiatric Interviewing: The Art of Understanding*. Philadelphia: W. B. Saunders, 1988.

2 | Appearance, Attitude, and Activity

The MSE begins as soon as the examiner sees the patient. Even before speaking, the astute examiner carefully notes the patient's appearance and may learn something about the patient's interactions with others, such as those in the waiting room. Close observation of the patient is continued throughout the interview, and the data obtained are summarized in the first section of the MSE report—the Appearance, Attitude, and Activity section (some shorten this heading to Appearance and Behavior). Many features of the patient's appearance and behavior that should be observed, including physical characteristics, nonverbal communications, and motor function, are reported in this section of the MSE.

It is important to be careful and nonjudgmental in the choice of words used to describe the patient's appearance and attitude. This is necessary both to be fair to the patient and to prevent embarrassment to the examiner if the MSE report is reviewed in an unforeseen venue, such as during litigation. The physician should avoid slang and prejudicial or prejorative terms. Careful attention to one's own attitude and word choice is recommended when describing age, sex, race, or other areas in which social bias may be encountered. Some terms used to describe appearance, activity, and attitude are part of our everyday vocabulary, whereas others are technical terms. Especially when using the vernacular, it is crucial to avoid judgmental words; for example, it is preferable to write "child-like" instead of "childish."

Appearance refers to the physical characteristics of the patient, including bodily habitus, physical disabilities or abnormalities, dress, grooming, and cleanliness. Appearance can be a clue to mood, rate of aging, cognitive state, self-awareness, presence of thought disorder, motor condition, and general physical health. *Attitude* refers to the patient's approach to the interview and interaction with the examiner (e.g., whether cooperative, hostile, facetious, or inappropriately familiar). The patient's attitude toward the interview and examination will affect the data elicited, as well as possibly presage the quality of future interactions and success of the therapeutic alliance. Attitude may change during the course of the interview as anxiety decreases (or increases) and as rapport with the examiner builds (or deteriorates, as can happen with paranoid patients). *Activity* refers to the level and quality of the patient's physical (or motor) movement. Activity levels and types are useful indicators of concurrent mood states or of physical problems. Some patients cannot sit still, whereas others barely move, and others move in abnormal ways. Abnormal activity and movements can be indicative of a neurologic problem, and they may suggest diagnostic possibilities that should be explored by the psychiatrist through performance of a neurologic examination.

Application

Appearance

A description of the patient's appearance is typically the first element of a mental status record. It consists predominantly of the examiner's impressions and observations of what the patient looks like, but, if applicable, can include comments on sounds or odors emanating from the patient. Elements of a thorough report of appearance are summarized in Table 2–1. Even a brief MSE should minimally (1) include comments about the level of consciousness and apparent age; (2) mention marked abnormalities in any of the other areas mentioned in Table 2–1; and (3) record any obvious physical findings or any particularly noticeable or striking identifying features (e.g., goiter, limp, jaundice, diaphoresis, large birthmark). This portion of the MSE is intended to allow a person reading the report to form an accurate mental image of the patient. For example, one may record the following:

This is a middle-aged white male who appears older than stated age, is dressed in pajamas, disheveled, and unshaven. He is jaundiced, has ascites, a red nose, and perinasal telangiectasias. He remained supine in his hospital bed throughout the interview and made very little eye contact with the examiner. He wheezed audibly. He manifested psychomotor retardation and asterixis.

LEVEL OF CONSCIOUSNESS
Level of consciousness, also known as *level of arousal*, describes the patient's overall wakefulness or arousal. During the psychiatric interview, normal individuals are awake and alert, attentive to the examiner, and responsive to stimuli. In the MSE, this normal condition is reported as being alert. Occasionally, patients

Table 2.1. Items commonly included
in MSE report of appearance

Level of consciousness
Apparent age
Position
Attire
Cleanliness and grooming
Eye contact
Evident physical abnormality
Other striking or bizarre features

will be overly alert, a state that is termed *hypervigilant* or *hyperaroused*. Hypervigilant individuals appear anxiously attentive, do not relax, frequently scan the room, and are easily startled. This condition can be caused by mania, anxiety, paranoia, and physical problems such as hyperthyroidism or ingestion of sympathomimetic drugs (cocaine, amphetamines, etc.). Often, patients are encountered who are subnormally alert. A variety of adjectives are used to describe such a state of decreased arousal, but there is no clear consensus on the precise definition of these terms or on the differences among them. In approximate order of increasing severity, these terms include *drowsy, lethargic, obtunded, stuporous,* and *comatose.* These must be differentiated from normal sleep, from which patients can be fully aroused. *Drowsiness* is more or less synonymous with sleepiness or hypersomnia and is characterized by mental slowing, yawning, poor energy, and a tendency to fall asleep when not stimulated. *Lethargy* and *obtundation* are states representing degrees of more marked drowsiness and low energy. At the mild end they merge with drowsiness, and at the severe end with stupor. Some use the word *stupor* interchangeably with coma, but stupor is an appropriate term for those patients who occasionally emerge into brief periods of wakefulness to speak in response to very loud noises or painful stimuli. *Coma* is a state of unconsciousness from which patients cannot be aroused, even by repeated or noxious stimulation. The term *clouding of consciousness* has been used to refer generically to all of these degrees of diminished alertness, but because of its nonspecificity it should be avoided. Sometimes one encounters difficult-to-characterize patients who look awake yet show no evidence of mental activity. An example of such a condition is a *persistent vegetative state*, which may last for years after a severe brain injury. Sleep–wake cycles are present, and the open eyes may follow moving objects, which may give an inaccurate impression of consciousness. However, the patient cannot otherwise respond to the environment, and mental activity appears to be entirely absent. Neurologic lesions that prevent motor or vocal expression may result in a state that appears similar to a persistent vegetative one, but in which the unfortunate victim presumably retains conscious intelligence. This has been described as the *locked-in syndrome.* *Akinetic mutism* or *coma vigile* are, similarly, terms to describe wakeful-appearing but unresponsive individuals; however, it appears that they have been used by different authors to describe patients with varying degrees of retained consciousness; hence using these terms risks ambiguity.

Decreased alertness is associated with sleep deprivation or can be a sign of an underlying physical disturbance, including drug intoxication (e.g., alcohol, barbiturates, sedative/hypnotics, antidepressants), cerebral edema, a postictal state, concussion, central nervous system infection, large or acute structural brain lesions, delirium, or myxedema. Particular attention should be given to historical or examination evidence of fluctuating levels of alertness (or fluctuating level of consciousness) that often signal the presence of delirium. Impaired consciousness/arousal necessitates careful exploration for its explanation, and may indicate a need for emergent diagnostic or therapeutic procedures.

ATTENTIVENESS TO THE EXAMINER

Patients normally attend to the examiner and are interested in the examination. Lack of insight, hostility, or apathy may be conveyed by the patient who is overtly bored and uninterested. *Distractibility* refers to the inability to screen out irrelevant stimuli, such as noises outside the room, which precludes focusing on the interview. (See discussion of attentional deficits in Chapter 6.) Distractibility occurs in attention deficit disorder, mania, and "organic" mental disorders including delirium. The capacity for attention and concentration should therefore be carefully assessed in distractible patients (see Chapter 6). *Internal preoccupation* is signaled by episodic inattentiveness to the interviewer whenever the patient becomes distracted by intrusive thoughts or hallucinations, as occurs in severe depression and in various psychotic disorders (see Chapter 5). Autistic patients may exhibit profound lack of interest in social interactions and ignore the examiner, being engaged instead in play with inanimate objects or in self-stimulatory behaviors.

AGE

To what extent does the patient appear his or her age? This is a judgment by the examiner based on factors such as hair-style and hair color, skin condition, vigor, mode of dress, and so on. When patients appear older than their actual age, it may indicate poor physical health due to medical illness, alcohol abuse, depression, or perhaps a life-style wrought with excessive hardships, such as homelessness. Premature graying or baldness may affect self-esteem. Some patients may purposely attempt to appear older or younger than they actually are—for example, an adolescent whose pseudomaturity is due to inadequate parenting, or the middle-aged person who cannot accept the aging process. A commonly used description is "appears stated age" or "appears older than (younger than) stated age." Alternatively, patients may be directly described as "prepubertal," "young adult," "elderly-appearing," and so on. Stated age refers to the presumed age of the patient, usually based on the age the patient reports. In some instances, however, the patient (e.g., one who is demented) may not know his or her age, and the examiner may have to estimate it or obtain this information from a reliable third party.

POSITION AND POSTURE

Position and posture of the patient should be observed at the beginning of and during the interview. *Position* refers to the location of the patient's body in space (lying, sitting, kneeling, etc.), whereas *posture* refers to the arrangement of the patient's body parts (e.g., slumped, cross-legged, leaning, arms akimbo, etc.).

Patients seen in a general hospital may be lying in bed, perhaps even in traction or in restraints. Whereas some may refuse to sit, it is most common for patients to be sitting. Posture and position should be observed, and any readily evident abnormality recorded—for example, if a patient is slouching, rigidly erect, lying on one side because of pain, wheelchair-bound, or with his or her back to the examiner. Keeping arms and hands tightly crossed against the body may indicate anxiety, whereas lounging with arms over the back of furniture suggests confidence or even arrogance. Every posture may have significance, particularly when integrated with other MSE information, such as affect and attitude. Posture and position are important nonverbal clues to the patient's mood. For example, slouching in a chair with head hanging and eyes downcast may depict dejection or despair.

An abrupt change in the patient's posture may reflect his or her underlying emotional response to the topic of conversation, and so should be noted. For example, a middle-aged man may be sitting in an open, seemingly confident posture until the topic is raised of a boss who passed him over for promotion, at which point he leans menacingly toward the examiner.

Attire and Grooming

Attire and grooming reflect socioeconomic status, occupation, self-esteem, interest in life, socialization, and the motivation or ability to present oneself in an appropriate way for the interview. Expectations for attire and grooming must be modified depending on the context of the examination; being unshaven, uncombed, and dressed in pajamas may be expected in medically ill inpatients but not in outpatients coming for elective evaluation. The examiner should note coiffure, cleanliness, nails, facial hair, clothing, and, if applicable, oral hygiene and body odor. Unkempt or unclean appearance may indicate depression, mania, schizophrenia, or organic mental disorder (e.g., dementia or delirium), or may be a signal that the patient has no interest in impressing the examiner or is resistant to the idea of seeing a psychiatrist. Bizarre makeup often indicates psychosis (e.g., lipstick smeared across lower face rather than lips alone). Fastidiously groomed persons may be obsessive-compulsive or narcissistic (though, of course, fastidiousness is not necessarily pathologic). Clothing that seems incongruous for gender may indicate sexual identity issues or even psychosis. Hair changes or baldness may reflect nutritional abnormalities, radiation or chemotherapy, or trichotillomania. Bizarre haircuts may reflect psychosis, and shaving the head sometimes precedes other self-destructive acts. Cigarette-induced yellow or brown discoloration and burns of the fingers are common among the chronically mentally ill, and are a clue to smoking habits and self care. Dirty bodies and soiled clothing are sometimes encountered in outpatient and emergency settings and generally indicate self-neglect (e.g., due to dementia or severe psychosis) or significant deprivation (e.g., homelessness).

Even in brief mental status write-ups, it is customary to make some notation about clothing, cleanliness, and kemptness. Commonly employed descriptors include *unkempt, disheveled,* or *neatly dressed.* One should note any peculiarities in this area, while avoiding a judgmental tone. For example, it would be appropriate to note, "Hair is oily and fingernails are long and dirty," or "The patient wore a green sock on one foot and no sock on the other," or "Clothing was threadbare and torn," but not appropriate to write "He looks like a hippie," or "Her clothing is cheap."

Eye Contact

The degree to which a patient makes eye contact with the examiner often indicates his or her level of comfort in the interview. Suspicious persons may avoid eye contact, as will those who are coy, or wishing to deny the situation or their emotions. In some cultures, such as Islamic, it is considered rude to make direct eye contact. Hostile patients may stare to unnerve the examiner, whereas confused or intellectually impaired patients may stare because of lack of self-awareness. Depressed patients often look downward. Hallucinating patients may look in unexpected directions in response to their own internally produced visual or auditory stimuli. In first encounters, it is usually appropriate to follow the patient's lead; for example, an examiner's fixed stare could unnerve the patient who is overtly avoiding eye contact.

Physical Characteristics

Striking physical characteristics such as tattoos, needle marks, scars from prior suicide attempts or self-mutilation (particularly common on the anterior forearms), skin lesions or discoloration, unusual facial markings, obesity or thinness, sweating, handicaps, and amputated limbs should be noted, in addition to the usual demographic descriptors such as race, skin color, and sex. If the nature of the unusual feature is unclear, it is much better to ask the patient about it than to ignore it out of social delicacy. The examiner should note any odors emanating from the patient, including that of alcohol, feces, or urine; those produced by medical causes (e.g., fetor hepatis, ketone breath, anaerobic cellulitis); or foul body odor from lack of bathing. These give obvious clues to the patient's physical condition and self-care. Clues to physical problems may be found in sounds made by the patient, such as wheezes, coughs, or teeth grinding.

Facial Expression

Certain facial expressions can also convey information about the patient's mood, although these may be culturally biased. Such expressions might include sad, happy, angry, surprised, bored, irritated, disgusted, confused, anxious, or pained. Patients with right hemispheric lesions may have impaired facial expression of their emotions and difficulty recognizing the meaning of the facial expressions of others.

Attitude

The patient's attitude is appraised in the relationship between the patient and the examiner and in the patient's reactions to the interview process. Attitude may influence the validity and content of information elicited during the interview. In addition, the patient's general attitude at the time of the initial examination may be a guide to his or her capacity to form a *therapeutic alliance* (i.e., work constructively with a therapist), which is important to treatment planning.

Information about the patient's attitude is based on a summary of observations made by the examiner in the course of the interview. Attitude includes facial expressions and posture, completeness of answers, tone of voice, willingness to cooperate, attentiveness, degree of evasiveness in responses, and the fantasies and wishes of the patient as they relate to the interview process. In the written MSE report, patients are described as "cooperative," or the ways in which they fall short of this description are documented (see Table 2–2). The general demeanor of the patient is his or her predominant attitude. Adjectives such as friendly, trusting, preoccupied, cooperative, suspicious, arrogant, sarcastic, facetious, flippant, guarded, vigilant, threatening, hostile, impatient, regressed, childlike, and so on, are useful descriptors of demeanor. *Cooperative* describes the individual who is alert and attentive, and tries to communicate relevant information to the examiner, including by answering questions.

The degree of politeness during the interview may range from obsequiousness to hostile resistance. Normal assertiveness (e.g., identifying a topic as painful or interrupting the interview to answer the telephone) should not be construed as a lack of cooperation. Lack of cooperation may reflect personality disturbance, distraction by physical or mental distress, impaired alertness, impaired attentiveness, impaired memory, psychopathology, disinhibited behavior, impaired judgment, anger, or inept or insensitive interviewing.

Table 2.2. Terms commonly used
to describe attitude toward MSE

Cooperative
Uncooperative
Hostile
Guarded
Suspicious
Regressed

The patient's approach and attitude toward the examiner and the interview context may be greatly affected by the circumstances of the examination. For example, one might expect more resistance during the initial evaluation of an involuntarily hospitalized patient than in the office-based interview of an outpatient who is known to the examiner. Regressed patients may revert to dependent behavior in which they rely on others to take care of them. For example, children experiencing stress as a result of parental divorce may no longer follow toilet training behaviors; and ill adults may adopt the "sick role" to receive special attention and dispensations from responsibilities as though they were children. A guarded patient avoids self-disclosing statements. A vigilant patient may be hyperalert, warily looking about the room. A suspicious patient not only avoids self-disclosure but may also question the examiner (instead of the reverse). A hostile patient may communicate anger by appearance, words, or deeds.

Resistance is the conscious or unconscious attempt by the patient to withhold information or affect from the examiner. In psychodynamic psychotherapy, the term resistance describes any attempt by the patient, subtle or overt, conscious or unconscious, to avoid the exploration of sensitive or conflicted material. Personality-disordered persons are often *manipulative* in order to achieve their own ends. For example, an antisocial patient often appears charming but may circumvent answering certain questions that would reveal illicit drug dealing or other illegal behaviors. A histrionic patient may be seductive toward the examiner as a way to gain control of the interview. Lavish praise for the examiner and statements demeaning of previous caregivers may confirm the examiner's own feelings but, especially during the initial interview, may represent the idealization and devaluation commonly seen in borderline personality disorders. *Splitting* is the term used to describe the inability of a person to recognize good and bad features simultaneously in another individual (or institution). Patients with borderline personality disorder may seem strikingly variable in their attitude toward the therapist because of splitting (see Chapter 7). They are felt to have difficulty tolerating mixed or ambiguous feelings and so vacillate between all-positive feelings (*idealization*) and all-negative feelings (*devaluation*). Patients with developmentally primitive personality disorders, such as borderline and narcissistic, may lump (i.e., split) clinicians into all-good or all-bad status, and thus may be uncooperative after deciding the psychiatrist is all bad.

The patient may bring feelings to the interview that relate to past personal or family experience with psychiatry, or the patient may be inexperienced with the actual practice of psychiatry. These feelings may cloud or interfere with compliance during the interview—that is, may lead to resistance. If the patient exhibits a negative attitude toward the examiner, this may need to be explored before continuing the interview, as it is likely to affect adversely the information-gathering efforts of the examiner. Hostility, suspiciousness, vigilance, and guardedness should be carefully noted by the examiner. These are all evidence of a poor alliance or rapport between patient and examiner. This might suggest that the information provided by the patient is unreliable or incomplete, or may even signal the need for steps to protect the examiner's safety. Concerns about confidentiality may underlie the patient's negative feelings, and this may also need to be discussed specifically with the patient. Patients may be reluctant to cooperate if they are concerned that sensitive material will be discovered by others from whom they wish to conceal it. Idealized and unrealistic fantasies from a prior psychiatric experience can also contribute to a patient's negative attitude, particularly if they are felt to have been unfulfilled. Comments such as "You are the only doctor who can help me—you're not like all the others" signal that the patient may be idealizing the current physician. Although this may at first seem complimentary, it will probably set up the examiner for failure in fulfilling all the patient's hopes, just as all the other clinicians have failed.

Examiners may gain useful information in asking questions to which they know the answer. For example, an examiner in possession of documentation of past hospitalizations after suicide attempts might nevertheless ask, "Have you ever tried to harm yourself?" Injudicious use of such an approach obviously may be unrewarding or irritating to the patient, but careful use may teach a lot about the patient's veracity, completeness, or memory. It also allows the patient to present his or her version of history obtained from third-party sources.

Activity

Descriptors of motor activity, in combination with posture and position, provide a visual image of how patients appear in real life. An individual's physical movements can reveal information about his or her mood, energy level, muscle strength, coordination, and attitude. The MSE should record abnormalities in the level of activity; any abnormal motor activity or behavior; and any excessive, repeated, or distinctive activity or behavior. The patient's level of activity can range from *hyperactivity* to *bradykinesia* (slow movement, as in parkinsonism), to virtually no movement, as in a comatose or catatonic patient.

MOVEMENT

Lack of movement localized to an individual body part may indicate paresis or paralysis. There may be facial and limb *paresis* (weakness) or *paralysis* in the brain-damaged individual, or *pseudoparalysis* in the conversion-disordered patient. In *cataplexy*, the patient experiences a sudden, involuntary, but temporary loss of muscle tone and may drop to the floor; in some cases, only certain body parts such as eyelids may lose muscle tone. Patients with other neurologic disorders such as myasthenia gravis and periodic paralysis may present with alterations in muscle strength or tone.

Akinesia refers to a patient's tendency toward lack of motion, generally of a body part, despite intact motor strength. *Hypokinesia* is a less severe manifestation of the same phenomenon. A time-lapse photograph of an akinetic or hypokinetic patient would show fewer accessory movements than in normals. *Bradykinetic* patients move, but execute movements much more slowly than normal. The presence of hypokinesia and/or bradykinesia is most suggestive of a parkinsonian syndrome, but may be seen also in extreme depression, catatonia, epilepsy, and in diseases affecting the supplementary motor cortex. These symptoms should prompt the examiner to seek other evidence of parkinsonism, such as a resting tremor (see below), decreased accessory movements, difficulty initiating or changing movement, festinating gait, or masked facies. A patient who is said to have decreased *accessory movements* lacks associated automatic movements; there is little or no arm swing when walking, and no gesticulation during speaking. Absence of arm swing while walking is a very common manifestation of the extrapyramidal side effects of antipsychotic drugs. In fact, its presence is evidence that the patient has complied with taking these medicines. Difficulty in initiating or changing movement can be observed when such patients rise from a chair and begin to walk; they may have to rock back and forth or push themselves out of the chair with their hands. Their gait may be hesitant, then improve after a few steps; but then these patients are unable to stop abruptly or to change direction. A *festinating gait* begins with small, slow initial steps and gradually accelerates as though the patient is propelled forward; thus the patient may have difficulty stopping.

Masked facies reflects bradykinesia or akinesia of the muscles of facial expression and of eye closure, resulting in a reduced or absent expression, and hence a relatively fixed, masklike facial appearance. This can be confused with *blunted affect* (see Chapter 3), especially because masked facies and blunted affect are likely to occur in schizophrenic patients who are treated with antipsychotic drugs (which cause parkinsonian side effects). In cases of uncertainty, treatment with antiparkinsonian medications may clarify the diagnosis.

Psychomotor retardation is quite similar to bradykinesia, and some use the terms interchangeably. Others reserve psychomotor retardation to describe physical slowing attributed to psychologic, as opposed to overtly physical, causes. Psychomotor retardation is seen in depression and dementia; this slowing of motor activity is often accompanied by slowed mentation, slowed speech, or *abulia* (reduced spontaneity and increased latency of speech and action, decreased response to stimuli, and accuracy but terseness in verbal output). Catatonia (see below) could be construed as an extreme form of psychomotor retardation. Catatonia may occur in schizophrenia, depression, mania, conversion disorder, and delirium. Catatonia and depression-induced psychomotor retardation should be distinguished from the physical causes of akinesia/hypokinesia/bradykinesia, including parkinsonism, coma, brainstem and mesial–frontal cerebrovascular accidents, hydrocephalus, hypothyroidism, and neuroleptic malignant syndrome.

Some children with attention deficit disorder and manic patients are hyperactive and may even be unable to sit in one place during the interview. Anxious persons are often restless as are persons who experience restless legs syndrome or neuroleptic-induced akathisia. *Restlessness* can be manifested by legs jiggling around and other fidgeting, and the patient may even ask, "Is the interview over yet?" Asking an akathitic patient to sit or stand still typically worsens his or her discomfort. *Psychomotor agitation* refers to a general increase in physical activity associated with psychiatric disorders, such as agitated depression, delirium, and mania. Hyperactivity may also be caused by a known physical factor, such as intoxication with a stimulant drug.

TREMOR

Tremors are oscillating movements occurring in a relatively consistent rhythm. Tremors are evident most frequently in distal body parts, particularly the hands, but can involve other body parts and are not infrequently asymmetric. Tremor is typically of greater amplitude during periods of stress, and is abolished by sleep. Tremor may be categorized according to the circumstances under which it occurs: when the affected body part is resting; during postural activities (e.g., maintaining arms extended forward while standing); during action (e.g., eating or writing); or with intention (e.g., when the patient is tested with the finger-to-nose maneuver). Tremors may occur in more than one of these situations or be atypical in other ways. If a tremor does not fit neatly with one of the descriptions below, it is best to describe it carefully in the written MSE, as opposed to trying to force an inaccurate fit with one of the standard categories of tremor.

Resting tremor is coarse and of low frequency (about 3–8 cycles per second) and is evident when the extremity is in an attitude of repose (e.g., a hand resting on the patient's lap). Resting tremor disappears temporarily during movement; consequently, even severe cases may interfere little with purposeful movements. A common resting tremor combines flexion–extension movements of the fingers with thumb movements that produce a "pill-rolling" action. Resting tremors are typically associated with parkinsonism (whether antipsychotic-drug-induced, postencephalitic, idiopathic, etc.) and may be seen in neuroleptic malignant syndrome, neurosyphilis, or Wilson's disease.

Postural and *action tremors* are absent when the body is relaxed, but present when the body is actively maintained in a given posture, such as with arms outstretched. Depending on their etiology, postural and action tremors may be of as low a frequency as resting tremors, but may range to 10 cycles per second and above. Common causes are benign familial ("essential") tremor, hyperthyroidism, drug toxicity (lithium, stimulants, antidepressants, bromide, bismuth), alcohol or sedative-hypnotic withdrawal, neurosyphilis, or anxiety. Though they are more commonly associated with resting tremor, neuroleptic-induced parkinsonism and idiopathic parkinsonism can produce action and postural tremors.

Intention tremor occurs during the most demanding phases of an action. For example, when patients are asked to extend an arm and alternatively touch their nose and the examiner's finger, intention tremor becomes particularly evident when they hone in on the target (i.e., their hand may coarsely shake in front of their nose). Intention tremor can interfere with fine motor movements, but it is not evident during rest or the maintenance of a stable posture. Intention tremor is caused by disease of the cerebellum or its connections; thus it may be evident with cerebellar or brainstem tumor or vascular accident, multiple sclerosis, Wernicke's encephalopathy, Wilson's disease, or certain drug intoxications (e.g., alcohol, sedatives, phenytoin).

CHOREOATHETOID MOVEMENTS

Athetoid movements are snakelike writhings of the tongue, face, or extremities. They are slow and twisting. *Choreiform movements* also can be writhing, but are usually coarser, jerkier, and more discrete than athetoid movements. They can be brief, involuntary movements that interrupt the situation in an inappropriate way. Neither athetosis nor chorea is as rhythmic and regular as are resting tremors. *Hemiballismus*, related to chorea but far rarer, is a more violent, flinging or flailing movement of an extremity, usually only on one side of the body. Hemiballismus, like chorea, may disappear at rest. Though hemiballismus and chorea are described separately, they often occur together. Because they may be a source of embarrassment, the patient may try to cover up choreiform or hemiballistic movements by completing the motions as seemingly purposeful actions, such as primping hair or straightening a shirt. *Choreoathetoid movements* (a term that encompasses both chorea and athetosis) can be seen in Huntington's disease, rheumatic fever (Sydenham's chorea), tardive dyskinesia, Wilson's disease, hepatic encephalopathy, treatment with dopamine agonists, aging (senile chorea), lithium toxicity, and a variety of less common disorders. Hemiballismus is typically a result of a brain infarction or hemorrhage involving the subthalamic nucleus of the brainstem.

Tardive dyskinesia, associated with chronic neuroleptic drug use, is an extremely important disorder in psychiatry. Its presence should be sought and documented in any individual at risk (e.g., those who have been exposed to antipsychotic drugs). Though there is often involvement of the extremities, or even trunk or diaphragm, tardive dyskinesia most commonly involves the face, especially the mouth and tongue. The movements can be gross and disfiguring but are more frequently subtle; thus the examiner is likely to miss them in the absence of specific observation or examination for tardive dyskinesia. Although characteristic choreiform movements can often be observed to occur spontaneously, they may be more evident if patients are asked to perform certain actions, such as walking, resting with arms supported, opening and closing the mouth, and protruding the tongue. Volitional movement of one area of the body may unmask or aggravate dyskinesia in the affected area; thus movements of the hands or fingers may become more apparent during ambulation, and movements of the tongue may be noted if the patient is instructed to open his or her mouth while performing fine hand manipulations. Tardive dyskinesia is often measured serially in order to track its progression or its response to therapeutic interventions. The Abnormal Involuntary Movement Scale (AIMS) is a commonly used instrument that permits quantification of the severity of dyskinesia (National Institute of Mental Health, 1976).

DYSTONIAS

Dystonia bears some relationship to choreoathetoid movements, but the dystonic movement or posture is sustained for a longer duration and is more likely than chorea or athetosis principally to involve large muscles of the torso. Dystonias are involuntary increases in muscle tone that result in sustained contortions that cause the patient to remain in a distorted position such as a flexed back or twisted neck. *Acute dystonias* are the type most frequently seen in the psychiatric population and are usually side effects of antipsychotic drugs. Common presentations include twisting of the neck and back, eyes rolling up under the upper eyelids (*oculogyric crisis*), rotation and tilting of the head (*torticollis*), or backward arching of the back and neck (*opisthotonos*). Tongue and throat muscles may be involved, leading to difficulty in talking, swallowing, or even breathing. Acute dystonias are usually promptly reversed by anticholinergic drugs or benzodiazepines, but are usually quite painful and/or frightening to the patient, and can be misleading to the examiner who mistakes them for mannerisms of schizophrenia (see below). Acute dystonias usually last from a few seconds to (untreated) over an hour. Acute dystonia should also be differentiated from tetany. The latter is a painful, cramplike spasm, often of a peripheral limb muscle, such as carpopedal spasm.

   Chronic dystonias are reversible but recurrent, whereas fixed dystonias are irreversible abnormalities of posture. *Blepharospasm*, or repeated spasmodic closure of the eyelids, is probably a localized tardive dystonia; however, tics or tardive dyskinesia can have a similar appearance. *Tardive dystonia* is quite similar to tardive dyskinesia, but the movements (such as facial grimaces) are more sustained (at least several seconds) and less jerky. In addition to antipsychotic medication toxicity, important causes of acute and chronic dystonias include Huntington's disease, parkinsonism, Wilson's disease, hypoxic brain damage, kernicterus, and Hallervorden–Spatz disease. Opisthotonos and tetany can be seen in *Clostridium tetani* poisoning; tetany is also associated with hypoparathyroidism and other causes of hypocalcemia, hyperventilation during panic attacks and other causes of alkalosis, and pregnancy.

AUTOMATIC MOVEMENTS

Automatic behavior or *automatisms* are unconsciously initiated, involuntary movements that may be simple or complex, are usually purposeless, and can appear bizarre. Consciousness is impaired during automatic activity; the patient is either unresponsive or overtly confused, and frequently remains confused temporarily even after the behavior abates. Typically the patient has no memory of the automatism, unless it is in repeating what has been described by others who have witnessed the automatism. Common simple automatisms include chewing, licking, lip smacking, or clumsy movements of hands or feet. More complex examples are walking from room to room, or pulling at clothing or buttons. Automatisms can even include such complex behaviors as undressing, or continuing driving. Purposeful, organized violence is not characteristic of automatisms, but during automatic behavior, such patients may confusedly push away or strike at someone attempting to restrain them. Automatisms are most suggestive of complex partial seizures, and the more complex behaviors are almost always manifestations of epilepsy. Simple automatic behaviors may occur in fugue states and catatonia.

TICS

Tics are involuntary movements or vocalizations that range from simple to complex. An individual tic, such as clearing of the throat, may appear purposeful. However, tics are distinguished by their repetitiveness and the patient's inability consistently to resist them. Tics can briefly be consciously suppressed, but usually this requires much effort and produces anxiety that is relieved when the tic occurs. Common simple tics are blinking, facial grimacing, neck jerks, shoulder shrugging, throat clearing, and jerking movements of extremities. Most patients have an individualized repertoire of tics limited to one to several stereotyped, repetitive movements. Tics can and do afflict individuals who are in apparently good psychiatric health. They emerge most frequently, though usually transiently, in prepubescent children. Tics have also been associated with obsessive-compulsive disorder, caffeinism and stimulant drug use, Tourette's disease, and postencephalitic states. Tourette's (or Gilles de la Tourette's) disease is among the most severe of tic disorders; as this disease progresses, the repertoire of physical and vocal tics and other repetitive behaviors and obsessions grows. Patients suffering from this syndrome may display compulsive repetition of their own words (*palilalia*), repetition of the words of others (*echolalia*), or vocalization of profanity and obscenities (*coprolalia*).

The term *stereotypy* (or *stereotyped behavior*) is sometimes used to refer to repeated purposeless behaviors not under voluntary control. As such, this term overlaps considerably with automatism and tic. To avoid ambiguity, the term stereotypy is best reserved for the description of nonvolitional repeated behaviors that are more complex than tics but (unlike automatisms) are not associated with alteration of consciousness as are automatisms. An example of a stereotypy might be the rocking of a child with pervasive developmental disorder.

MANNERISMS

Mannerisms are consistent, characteristic, distinctive, apparently purposeful, highly stylized ways of doing things. They may seem very exaggerated or bizarre, as in schizophrenia. For example, a patient may habitually pirouette counterclockwise before sitting. Unlike complex tics, stereotypies, and automatisms, mannerisms are largely under voluntary control. Unlike automatisms, mannerisms are not accompanied by altered consciousness.

COMPULSIONS

Compulsions can be considered a subset of mannerisms: Any odd and repetitive complex behavior is a mannerism and may be a compulsion. *Compulsions* are actions that parallel obsessions and may be the motoric product of similar thoughts and urges as obsessions. Like obsessions, they are unwanted and ego-dystonic. They are often recognized by the patient as unreasonable; and attempts to voluntarily stop or suppress them are unsuccessful. During temporary suppression of compulsions, the patient grows anxious, and the anxiety is relieved by succumbing to performance of the compulsive act. The compulsive act is stereotyped (i.e., it is the same act over and over), often ritualistic (i.e., it is performed in the same manner each time), and often quite trivial. Common compulsive rituals include repetitive hand-washing, checking that the gas stove is turned off, or that the doors are locked. Other compulsions are completely idiosyncratic and appear to be mannerisms to the casual observer (e.g., an odd stereotyped behavior every time one enters a room, such as always making one clockwise circle), but in fact are performed to repress anxiety. Apparently goal-directed and potentially destructive behaviors (gambling, fire-setting) might also be compulsions. The urge or need to perform a compulsive act repeatedly forces itself into the patient's consciousness, which some refer to as an impulsive obsession. Very frequently, the compulsive act is directly linked to an obsession; for example, those persons who are obsessed or preoccupied with exposure to germs may wash themselves excessively after touching anything that is conceivably contaminated. Others may compulsively perform some action (e.g., making the sign of the cross) every time the obsessive thought occurs. These actions occur almost automatically and are also known as compulsive rituals or ritualistic behaviors. (See also mannerisms and automatic behaviors.)

Those compulsive actions that result in behaviors that are consequential for these patients or for those around them have special clinical importance. Some of these may be true compulsions; alternatively, they may be *habits*, which are usually less severe than compulsions and can be consciously suppressed. Drug and alcohol addictions may have a compulsive component that could be consciously suppressed if motivation were adequate; however, the negative consequence of withdrawal symptoms may reduce willingness to abstain. Many pleasurable behaviors have a compulsive aspect (e.g., substance abuse, overeating, gambling, voyeurism), but because some of these behaviors are illegal, the patient may overemphasize the uncontrollability of the acts. A truly compulsive impulse is irresistible; its psychologic purpose is to dispel anxiety, and it can be resisted only briefly and uncomfortably.

There are many habitual behaviors that have been at times labeled compulsions; frequently these are named with suffixes *-mania* or *-philia*. Most people who engage in habitual behaviors are not truly compulsive; the term compulsion should be used only if the impulse is repetitive, ritualistic, and essentially irresistible. A full list of such items is beyond the scope of this book but can be found in other reference manuals, such as the *Psychiatric Dictionary*. Some examples include *kleptomania* (stealing), *pyromania* (fire-setting), *trichotillomania* (hairpulling), *necrophilia* (sexual attraction to corpses), *pedophilia* (sexual attraction to children), *nymphomania* (a female's compulsion to engage in sexual intercourse), and *satyriasis* (a male's compulsion to engage in sexual intercourse).

In screening for compulsions, patients can be asked if they have any eccentricities or habits. If an affirmative reply is suggestive of a compulsion or a possible compulsion is observed, patients should be asked whether they are aware of the behavior, whether it has happened in other circumstances, and whether they would like to stop doing it but cannot. If the answer is yes to all of those questions, the behavior is probably a compulsion, and further inquiry should be made regarding the accompanying thought content and the presence of any obsessions. Compulsions are characteristic of obsessive-compulsive disorder, but occur in the context of other psychiatric illnesses, as well as in certain neurologic conditions, notably Gilles de la Tourette's disorder. The diagnostic significance of these symptoms is discussed in more detail under Obsessions and Preoccupations, in Chapter 5. If the mannerism occurs in the presence of a clouded consciousness or the patient is unaware of it, it is not likely a compulsion, and questioning should instead be directed to the presence of a partial complex seizure disorder.

If a possible compulsion is noted, questioning should clarify if the action is unwanted and ego-dystonic, if the patient has tried to stop it, and in what way and how severely it affects the patient's life.

OTHER MOTOR ABNORMALITIES

Perseveration is an incapacity for or difficulty in shifting from one task to another. It is typically verbal, as in inappropriate repetition of a word or phrase (also known as *verbigeration*), but also physical (*motor*), such as repeatedly performing a previously requested task in the interview while failing to initiate a more recently requested task. Perseveration implies dysfunction of the prefrontal cortex; it is seen in head injuries, strokes, tumors, dementias, or other degenerative diseases affecting this brain area. Perseveration is also encountered in schizophrenia, especially in catatonic patients. Perseveration and verbigeration can be confused with automatisms, but are distinguished by the absence of alteration of consciousness and by the overall clinical context.

Posturing refers to sustaining an apparently purposeless, nonresting position, such as with one arm in the air for minutes to days. In *catatonia*, patients may hold a position for hours without moving. Posturing also occurs in complex partial seizures. *Echopraxia* is the uncontrolled mimicking of another's movement and posture (as opposed to perseveration, the repeating of one's own movements). In *catalepsy* or *waxy flexibility*, a limb or other body part is kept in any position, even ridiculous, in which another person places them. Hence, the examiner can mold the patient's posture, as if with a soft wax doll. Although one classically thinks of catatonic behavior as meaning immobility, catatonic patients can have hyperactive episodes that are referred to as *catatonic excitement*. The excited catatonic may display remarkable examples of many motor abnormalities including mannerisms, verbigeration, motor perseveration, and echolalia. This state of hyperactivity is a potentially dangerous condition if the agitation is suddenly and uncontrollably expressed. Catatonic symptoms such as posturing or catalepsy are most classically associated with schizophrenia. However, the syndrome and symptoms are nonspecific and have been reported in bipolar psychoses, hysteria, hypnosis, dementia, and physical brain disturbances such as epilepsy or certain drug intoxications.

OTHER MOTOR EXPRESSIONS

In addition to the above-mentioned aberrations of movement, the examiner should note actions or movements that, while not necessarily abnormal in themselves, are meaningful, distinctive, or repetitive. These include pacing, hand wringing, fist clenching or shaking, grimacing, throwing things, pounding and assaultive behaviors, head banging, obscene gestures, and so forth. Unlike most other movement disorders discussed, these are more or less under volitional control. Sleepwalking may be reported by nursing staff or family members; it is a *parasomnia* associated with deep sleep, so it is usually not evident during psychiatric examination.

Finally, physical manifestations of emotional expression are also relevant. These include crying, laughing, screaming, sniffling, whistling, grunting, and singing. These expressions may be appropriate or may be incongruent to the context, which is important to note. For example, crying when sad is congruent; crying when happy is not.

Unfortunately, comments regarding motor behavior and abnormal movement are frequently not included in psychiatric reports, perhaps reflecting a tendency to focus on mental functions at the expense of their physical expressions. The importance of abnormalities in this area cannot be overstated: they are key clues to physical etiologies of illness and/or psychotropic drug toxicity. If an observed unusual behavior does not fit well within a classification (e.g., resting tremor) described above, it is best to describe the signs and symptoms of the behavior with as much elaboration as is required to clearly depict them. In the absence of an abnormality, it is often worthwhile to record the negative, such as "motor activity normal, no movement disorder." This provides a baseline for future exams.

Beyond recording motoric abnormalities, the examiner can think carefully about them in formulating diagnostic hypotheses; this in turn will shape the questions posed in completing a history and MSE. For example, the observation of a grimacing tic should remind the examiner that tics can be associated with obsessive-compulsive disorder, Tourette's disease, and stimulant abuse, and therefore prompt questioning to rule in or out each of these disorders.

Definitions

Abulia   Decreased activity due to lack of ability or power to execute action, despite a desire to do so. This is often associated with slowing or increased latency of mentation and speaking. Abulic patients have been described as inert, uncaring, and undriven; consequently, this condition may resemble depression, but abulic patients will typically not cry or report feeling sad. Abulia is most often seen in schizophrenics or brain-injured patients with injuries to frontal lobes or basal ganglia. Abulic patients are slow in performing simple cognitive tasks, such as counting backward.

Agitation   A general term used to describe a condition in which a person seems emotionally distressed, cannot sit still or attend, and gives evidence of heightened tension. Agitation may result from a wide variety of underlying conditions, including acute grief, generalized anxiety, heart or thyroid disease, medical crisis, drug intoxication or withdrawal, cognitive dysfunction, mania, and psychosis.

Aggression   Behaviors or attitudes that reflect rage, hostility, and the potential for physical or verbal destructiveness. Unlike assertiveness, which is a socially appropriate means of limit-setting and self-definition, aggression is the expression of negative affect meant to assault, harm, or manipulate another person, animal, or object in some way. Aggression may be volitionally planned and/or due to poor impulse control. Aggressive behavior may occur in antisocial and borderline personality-disordered patients and in frontal lobe-impaired persons, in part related to an inability to empathize with others; in demented, psychotic, or delirious patients who erroneously perceive other persons as intending to harm them; in brain-injured patients who have lost impulse control or have poor social judgment; or in conduct- and intermittent explosive-disordered children. In conduct, borderline personality, and antisocial disorders, aggression is usually volitional and intentional, whereas in other disorders it is more related to thought disorder or to organically reduced impulse control.

Akathisia A feeling of motoric restlessness, particularly of the legs, usually a side effect of neuroleptic medication (i.e., antipsychotic drugs). Strictly speaking, akathisia is a subjective experience, and therefore, its diagnosis is based on patients' reports. However, patients with akathisia may appear to tremble nervously, shake their legs (even when sitting), or keep getting up to walk around. Attempts to remain still are likely to increase discomfort. Akathisia should be differentiated from anxiety, psychotic agitation, agitated depression, and restless legs syndrome.

Akinesia A marked reduction in accessory motor activity (e.g., arms swinging while walking) and in normal automatic movements (e.g., blinking, swallowing, periodic postural adjustment). There may be an associated slowing of mentation (abulia). It is associated with psychotic states, extreme depression, catatonia, epilepsy, and movement disorders such as parkinsonism (including that induced by antipsychotic drugs). Lesions of the supplementary motor cortex and hydrocephalus can produce akinesia and mutism. Differentiate akinesia from paralysis.

Apathy A lack of emotions or desire, a feeling of uninvolvement, or not caring. The outward manifestation of apathy may be confused with that of abulia (see above). Apathy occurs most often in depression and schizophrenia (see Chapter 3).

Athetoid Movements Abnormal movements that are slow, writhing, involuntary, and involving the extremities (e.g, fingers, hands, and sometimes toes or tongue). These are often described as snakelike.

Automatic Movements Involuntary movements that occur in the setting of altered consciousness; also termed automatisms. These may occur in psychotic states including catatonia and in hysterical fugue states, but are most suggestive of complex partial or absence seizures. These movements vary widely in character and complexity, from bizarre, purposeless movements to complex behaviors. If automatisms originate in one epileptic focus, the clinical presentation is often consistent from one episode to the next. Common epileptic automatisms include lip-smacking and swallowing (in complex partial seizures), and rhythmic rapid eye-blinking (in absence seizures).

Bradykinesia A slowing of motor activity, as though one is in slow motion. It is common in extrapyramidal syndromes such as parkinsonism (whether due to idiopathic disease, other degenerative disorders, or medication), as well as in schizophrenia and major depression.

Catalepsy The maintenance of certain bodily positions or postures for prolonged periods of time. Vital signs (pulse and respirations) may also be slowed (see Waxy flexibility, below). It is often associated with catatonic states, such as in schizophrenia. Do not confuse with cataplexy.

Cataplexy A temporary state of sudden involuntary muscle relaxation causing loss of postural muscle tone, in the setting of intact consciousness. The outcome ranges from falling down to only eyelid closure. It occurs in association with narcolepsy and is related to rapid eye movement (REM) sleep that abnormally intrudes into wakefulness. It is often precipitated by laughter, fright, or emotional stress. Cataplexy is not in itself evidence of a major psychiatric disorder.

Catatonia A severe, psychotic disturbance of motor function. It is usually manifested by markedly decreased activity, but may entail hyperactivity ("catatonic excitement"), with alternation between these states. In the hypoactive state the person is immobile and maintains peculiar postures for long periods of time (see Catalepsy, above). The limbs are either rigid or flexible when moved passively by the examiner. Patients may be echopraxic (see this section) and are generally mute, though they may be echolalic or have verbigeration (see Chapter 4). Automatisms and extreme bradykinesia can occur, as well as grimacing and staring. Catatonic patients may be excessively excited underneath the emotionally unresponsive and motorically statuesque exterior; they may become combative. In catatonic excitement, patients show a markedly high degree of activity which is usually purposeless and associated with abnormalities such as grimacing, posturing, or automatisms. It is a relatively rare condition, most often seen in schizophrenics, manics, depressives, and other psychotics. The differential diagnosis of catatonia includes partial complex seizures, viral encephalitis, severe parkinsonism, neuroleptic malignant syndrome, delirium, lesions of the mesial frontal region, and neurosyphilis.

Cogwheel rigidity A finding of involuntary resistance to passive flexion/extension and pronation/supination (e.g., at the elbow) or rotational movements around a joint (e.g., at the wrist). A ratcheting sensation (of alternating muscle tension and relaxation) is felt by the examiner. This characterizes the rigidity of Parkinson's disease and, as such, often accompanies bradykinesia. It also occurs as an extrapyramidal side effect from antipsychotic drugs. It is distinguished from lead-pipe rigidity (as occurs in the neuroleptic malignant syndrome) in that the latter is extreme stiffness without the ratcheting.

Choreiform movements Irregular, involuntary movements of face, limb, or trunk muscles, which are faster, jerkier, and more discrete than athetoid movements. They are thought to reflect basal ganglia dysfunction and can be a manifestation of basal ganglia infarction, tumors, or calcification. They may occur concurrently with athetoid movements. Hemiballismus is a related but more extreme movement disorder. Patients may try to cover up these choreiform movements by continuing the abnormal motion into a seemingly purposeful motion, such as grooming their hair or primping their clothes. The irregularity of these movements helps to distinguish them from the rhythmic tremor of Parkinson's disease. Choreiform movements are seen in tardive dyskinesia, Huntington's chorea, Sydenham's chorea, advanced age, and toxicity from certain drugs (e.g., amphetamines, phenytoin, estrogens, dopamine agonists, and lithium).

Coma Profound unconsciousness with loss of voluntary activity and communication. Patients may appear to be asleep, although they cannot be aroused. It is usually due to severe bihemispheric or brainstem reticular formation dysfunction, on a structural or metabolic basis. It must be differentiated from an hysterical condition, catatonic stupor, or the "locked-in syndrome" associated with pontine tegmental lesions. In locked-in syndrome, the patient is awake and aware but unable to activate muscles other than those controlling vertical eye movements and/or eye closure.

Compulsion Unwanted, ego-dystonic impulse to perform certain motor behaviors. The patient usually realizes that the behavior is unreasonable, but can suppress it only temporarily and at the expense of increasing anxiety. Common compulsions involve washing or checking. Compulsions often accompany obsessions and may be directly linked to them (see Chapter 5).

Disinhibited behavior The term often used broadly to refer to poor self control or loss of the capacity to resist unacceptable impulses. More narrowly, it refers to characteristic and socially inappropriate speech and behavior sometimes seen in patients with severe dysfunction of the frontal lobes; similar phenomena are described in schizophrenia, ethanol intoxication, and sometimes in the context of lesions of the brainstem or thalamus. These patients display exaggerated and inappropriate rudeness, candor, lewdness, profanity, jocularity, sexual behavior or preoccupation, and/or public undressing or voiding. Childish joking or pranks are known as *witzelsucht*. (Refer to the discussion of Judgment in Chapter 7.)

Dystonia An episode of involuntary increased tone in a muscle or group of muscles that occurs rarely in parkinsonism and, more frequently, as an extrapyramidal side effect of antipsychotic drugs. These commonly cause immobility or a thick feeling of the mouth or tongue. A potentially dangerous form is laryngospasm because it threatens the airway. More severe varieties include unilateral spasm of the sternocleidomastoid muscle with rotation and/or tilting of the head (*torticollis*), eyeballs rolling upward, usually accompanied by extension of the neck (*oculogyric crisis*), or bending over backward such that the back of the head approaches the legs (*opisthotonos*).

Echopraxia Involuntary repetition and imitation of another person's (e.g., the examiner's) movements, inappropriate to the situation. It is also termed *echokinesis*. It is seen in catatonia, tic disorders, and sometimes in partial complex seizures, frontal lobe damage, and dementias.

Extrapyramidal side effects The pyramidal tracts of the lower brainstem (medulla oblongata) contain fibers of the corticospinal tract—that is, axons of upper motor neurons of the voluntary motor pathway. Clinicians have consequently adopted the term *extrapyramidal system* to group all the other (involuntary) central neural structures and pathways subserving movement, tone, and posture. Among other things, the so-called extrapyramidal system includes elements of the cerebellum, basal ganglia, and brainstem. In psychiatric patients, the term extrapyramidal side effects (often abbreviated EPS or EPSE) almost always refers to drug (usually antipsychotic)-induced abnormalities of the extrapyramidal system, commonly but not of necessity resembling idiopathic Parkinson's disease. EPS subsumes tremor, bradykinesia, cogwheeling, paratonia (diffuse muscle stiffness), dystonia, and akathisia (see parkinsonian movements in this section). It is generally preferred to list individually the specific extrapyramidal symptom or sign—for example, resting tremor, akathisia, oculogyric crisis, and so on.

Eye contact Normally persons comfortably conversing with each other look at each other often, but without staring. Depressed, socially awkward (e.g., avoidant personality disorder, right-hemisphere learning-disabled patients), paranoid, or schizophrenic persons may avoid eye contact with others, instead looking downward or away. Manic or aggressive patients may stare excessively, making the other person feel uncomfortable. Catatonic patients often stare, as do patients during absence seizures.

Guarded behavior Behavior or attitude in which the patient attempts to conceal information and/or is hesitant to reveal particular details for fear of imagined or realistic repercussions. This behavior is inferred by the examiner. It may occur in the context of suspiciousness, psychosis, or paranoia; and in antisocial personality-disordered patients who are manipulative and trying to hide self-incriminating information.

Hyperactivity Excessive motoric activity which may or may not be associated with mental changes. Patients frequently appear distractible and are unable to sit calmly in one place and, instead, walk or run around, keep changing position, or keep doing things. Akathisia is usually associated with treatment with antipsychotic drugs or with Parkinson's disease, and is less likely to be associated with purposeful behaviors than is hyperactivity and is more likely to be accompanied by subjective anxiety. Hyperactivity involves gross body movements, not simply restless fidgeting. Associated with mania, attention deficit disorder, catatonic excitement, drug intoxication or withdrawal, and mental retardation.

Lead pipe rigidity Markedly increased muscle tone and resistance to passive movement independent of the direction of movement. The patient is almost as stiff as a board. In addition, during movement of an extremity, the muscle tone is smooth and consistent during all degrees of motion; that differentiates it from *cogwheel rigidity* in which the tension alternates in a ratcheting fashion, and from *paratonia* in which there is a momentary reduction in muscle tone if direction is suddenly reversed. Lead pipe rigidity may indicate brain damage, neuroleptic malignant syndrome, or acute withdrawal from dopaminergic medications in a parkinsonian patient.

Manipulative Attitude or behavior in which one exploits, outsmarts, or subtly coerces another person in order to gain advantage, maintain control, or get one's own way. This behavior is inferred by the examiner. It is an indirect and psychologically "immature" manner of relating to another person. Sometimes the feelings of others are manipulated, including managing to get the other person to feel guilty, in order to achieve one's own wishes. At times it is more overt—for example, threatening to kill oneself in order to gain admission to the hospital or to have a family member agree to something that he or she ordinarily would not. The person being manipulated usually feels angry once the manipulation has been accurately perceived for what it is. It is common in many types of personality disorders (e.g., borderline, histrionic, and antisocial) and in normal children (see Chapter 7).

Mannerism A peculiar and repetitive body movement or action that appears bizarre to the observer because it is exaggerated or out of context and does not resemble known types of involuntary movements. Tics and mannerisms can sometimes be distinguished only by history, as mannerisms can be ticlike. Mannerisms are presumed to be more volitional than tics, but this may be difficult to ascertain. A mannerism may involve a particular posture, gait, or motion such as a hip wiggle. It may have meaning to the patient.

Motor perseveration Deficient capacity to shift from one motor behavior to another. This may be spontaneously evident, or may be observed in the patient's difficulty in switching from one assigned task to another, such as difficulty stopping performance of the finger-to-nose maneuver.

Parkinsonian movements   Involuntary movements due to dysfunction of the basal ganglia, including resting tremor, cogwheeling, muscular rigidity, masked facies, bradykinesia, and festinating gait. These signs occur in parkinsonism and other extrapyramidal disorders such as progressive supranuclear palsy; as side effects of antipsychotic medications; following brain anoxia or carbon monoxide poisoning; in encephalitis and neurosyphilis; or after exposure to carbon disulfide, manganese, or MPTP (an opiate drug that is a chemical intermediate synthesized during illegal meperidine production).

Psychomotor retardation   Slowing of body movements secondary to psychic dysfunction. It is typically accompanied by hypokinesia or akinesia. It is seen in delirium, major depression, drug intoxication or withdrawal, hypothyroidism, dementia, and schizoaffective disorder.

Regressed behavior   A deterioration to a behavior that is psychosocially less mature (developmentally speaking) than expected by the individual's age or stage of life. The patient may appear childlike, with increased dependence on others. Indecision, fear of being alone, petulance, decreased self-care, or incontinence may be seen in regressed individuals. Temporary regression, especially if not severe, may be a normal occurrence when one becomes physically ill and needs to be taken care of. Responsibilities, actions, and communications normally expected from adults are forsaken. It may occur in elderly demented persons and in schizophrenics.

Resistance   Unconscious or subconscious opposition to attempts by others to help the patient or to bring into the patient's awareness information or ideas that are conflictual and uncomfortable. This can be frustrating for the clinician who may perceive it as inertia. The patient may distrust the clinician or fear embarrassment, and so withhold information or not fully cooperate with treatment or evaluation efforts.

Splitting   A psychologic defense mechanism in which other persons and things are viewed in extremes, without the ability to consider compromise or to integrate seemingly conflicting information into a whole (see Chapter 7). Things are either "black" or "white," or "good" or "bad." The patient alternatively idealizes or denigrates the same person, or splits groups of others (family, hospital staff, etc.) into good guys and bad guys. Outward manifestations of splitting may be inferred by the patient's attitude or behaviors during the examination.

Stereotypy   A repetitive, purposeless movement. This term overlaps considerably with (and some use it synonymously with) tic, automatism, and mannerism. In this broad sense it refers to repetitive idiosyncratic movements that are adequately consistent to characterize or describe the patient, and are presumed to be nonvolitional or at least poorly controlled by the patient. In a more narrow sense, it is used to describe behaviors such as the rocking or head banging of autistic children. In this narrower sense, stereotypies are more complex than simple tics and, unlike automatisms, occur without concomitant alteration of consciousness.

Suspiciousness   Distrust of others or their intentions; being more sensitive to or vigilant regarding others. It is not as severe as paranoia or as tightly held as a delusion, and may be founded or unfounded.

Tics   Abnormal sudden, repetitive, stereotyped jerky movements of eyes, vocal organs, face, extremities, or trunk. Vocal tics may be verbal utterances or gutteral sounds (see Chapter 4). Tics typically occur many times during each day, but generally decrease during sleep, and may increase with stress. Tics include eye blinking, grimacing, biting, kicking, and coughing. Tics may be the result of Gilles de la Tourette's disease, anxiety, stimulant use, stroke, encephalitis, or Huntington's chorea and may be transient during childhood. Although considered involuntary, patients can often suppress them for brief periods of time in social situations, but may feel compelled to produce them and experience anxiety and discomfort while suppressing them.

Tremors   Rapidly alternating movements of the extremities, trunk, head and neck, tongue, or lips which occur when the limb or trunk is at rest, held in a posture, or executing intentional motions. This shakiness can be either fine (subtle) or coarse (larger movements). Tremors may be of physiologic frequency (roughly 15 cycles per second), but are often slower. Types of pathologic tremors are postural (action), intention, and resting. A "pill-rolling" resting tremor is said to occur when the patient appears to be rolling a pill between his or her thumb and fingers and is seen classically in parkinsonian patients. Tremors are seen with anxiety, delirium, drug intoxication and withdrawal, alcohol withdrawal, cerebellar disease, hyperthyroidism, hypothermia, parkinsonism, lithium use or toxicity, cyclosporine treatment, familial tremor, and panic disorder.

Vigilance   Sustained attention to external stimuli. Anxious or paranoid persons or those expecting something important to happen may be hypervigilant. Excessive vigilance may interfere with normal sleep. Vigilance is reduced in some confusional states and in the hemispatial neglect syndrome, in which the patient fails to attend adequately to stimuli in one hemispace (usually the left).

Viscosity   The "gluey" interictal behavior of some patients with temporal lobe epilepsy, including interpersonal clinginess, difficulty breaking conversations, and excessive talking. Viscosity is possibly more likely to be associated with left-sided seizure focus.

Waxy flexibility   Also called *cerea flexibilitas* or *catalepsy*. The patient's posture is held in a fixed position for a prolonged period of time, even in odd positions such as standing with arms extended like a tree. There is usually resistance to the examiner's attempts to alter the positions.

References

Adams, R. D., and Victor, M. *Principles of Neurology*, 4th edition. New York: McGraw Hill, 1989.

Kaplan, H. I., and Sadock, B. J. *The Comprehensive Textbook of Psychiatry*, 5th edition. Baltimore: Williams and Wilkins, 1989.

Klawans, H. L. Recognition and diagnosis of tardive dyskinesia. *Journal of Clinical Psychiatry* 4: 3–7, 1985.

Lishman, W. A. *Organic Psychiatry: The Psychological Consequences of Cerebral Disorder*, 2nd edition. Oxford: Blackwell Scientific Publications, 1987.

National Institute of Mental Health. Abnormal involuntary movement scale (AIMS). In *Early Clinical Drug Evaluation Assessment Manual*, edited by W. Guy. Rockville, Md.: U.S. Department of Health and Human Services, 1976, pp. 534–7.

Plum, F., and Posner, J. *The Diagnosis of Stupor and Coma*, 3rd edition. Philadelphia: F. A. Davis, 1980.

Rowland, L. (ed.). *Merritt's Textbook of Neurology*, 8th edition, Philadelphia: Lea & Febiger, 1989.

3 | Mood and Affect

Mood and affect are terms used to describe emotional or feeling states. A disturbance of mood or affect is the key feature of some of the most common and important psychiatric disorders, including depression and mania.

A *mood* is a person's predominant internal feeling state at a given time. Everyone can be said to be in some particular mood, usually determined by disposition and circumstances. In a mental status report, mood should be empirically described. Virtually no particular mood is necessarily abnormal or pathologic; rather, mood must be assessed in the context of the patient's entire history and MSE. This chapter focuses on terminology that is used to describe various aspects of mood.

Affect is the external and dynamic manifestation of a person's internal emotional state, and hence is present in all individuals. It may or may not match a person's stated mood. Affect is judged in terms of its type, intensity, range, variability, and degree of correspondence to the content of conversation. Normal individuals demonstrate a variety of emotions, of variable intensity, that usually match and change in accordance with the thoughts and feelings being verbally expressed.

Mood and affect are sometimes difficult to distinguish from each other. The beginning examiner can avoid confusion by defining mood as the patient's subjective description of his or her feeling state, while defining affect as the objectively observable manifestations of the feeling state(s). However, some psychiatrists rely not on this subjective/objective dichotomy but rather on the aspect of changeability to differentiate mood from affect. In that paradigm, mood is a consistent, sustained feeling state, whereas affect is the moment-to-moment expression of feelings. Both of these conventions can be applied.

Two important psychiatric disorders involve a disturbance of mood or affect as their main feature: depression and mania. In *depressive disorders* the predominant emotion is usually dysphoria or melancholia. The patient describes feeling sad, blue, low, and unable to experience pleasure. In *manic disorders* the predominant emotion is elation, with grandiosity, increased energy, and social inappropriateness. However, in some manic patients the predominant mood is irritability, and they present as being angry or petulant.

Disturbances of mood and affect may be present in or occur concurrently with psychiatric disorders other than the affective disorders—for example, schizophrenia, delirium, dementia, personality disorders, drug and alcohol dependence, anxiety disorders, and adjustment disorders—and in stress reactions in

previously healthy individuals. Medical diseases such as hyper- and hypothyroidism, cancer, parkinsonism, brain tumors, multiple sclerosis, systemic lupus
erythematosus, and epilepsy may present with disturbances of mood and affect.
Many medications, such as corticosteroids, alpha-methyldopa, reserpine, cal-
cium channel blockers, antiviral agents, and phenobarbital can cause changes in
mood.

Application

Mood

The patient's current mood is assessed throughout the course of the interview. In
the absence of a significant provocation, mood is normally a relatively sustained
and predominant emotional state that is more likely to vary over hours or days
than over minutes or seconds. Usually a variety of emotional expressions, particularly nonverbal ones, are exhibited during the course of an interview. This
observed mood and its variability constitute affect and will be discussed below.

The most straightforward approach in describing mood is simply to equate it
with whatever the patient reports as his or her subjective emotional state. This
works best when the patient is articulate and consistent and when his or her
verbal report matches the nonverbal expression. Patients should be encouraged
to describe their emotional state in their own words. Mood is often spontaneously reported by the patient; in fact, a mood disturbance is a common reason
to seek professional consultation. If not spontaneously reported, the examiner
must explicitly ask about mood, progressively using more directive questions as
needed. Open-ended questions like "How have you been feeling lately?" or "How
do you feel right now?" should be used initially. Patients should be encouraged to
elaborate on their responses, with particular attention to whether their current
mood is typical for them and what the intensity of their emotions is. The use of
synonyms and qualifiers should be encouraged to ensure mutual understanding
of a given word. For example, patients may use the word depressed for apathetic,
nervous for tremulous, or hypertensive for excited. To gauge the intensity of
feelings, the examiner might ask a depressed patient: "What do you mean by the
word 'depressed'?" or "What is it like to feel depressed?" or "How depressed are
you?" or "Where would you rate yourself on a scale of one to ten, if one is the
worst you have ever felt and ten is the best?" or "Is being depressed the same as
being sad (or without energy, not caring, down in the dumps, angry, etc.)?"

If patients will not spontaneously describe their mood, prompting questions
may be developed, with regard to the patient's affect or thought content. Appropriate use of statements like "That must make you very angry" or "You look quite
sad when you talk about that" may both communicate empathy and stimulate

comment from the patient. If open-ended questions do not succeed, direct questions ("Are you feeling remorseful?") should be employed.

In certain cases, describing mood may be particularly challenging for the patient and examiner. The *alexithymic* patient has great difficulty putting emotions into words, and may even fail to understand questions such as "How do you feel?" Psychotic patients may describe their mood in incongruous or neologistic terms ("I'm bum-fried"). Personality-disordered patients may give inconsistent descriptions of their mood and may have more changeable moods than most people ("moody"). Mood cannot be adequately ascertained in noncommunicative patients, such as in elective mutism and locked-in syndrome. In these difficult cases, the written report should describe both what is observed and the limitations or inconsistencies of the findings.

In the MSE report, mood is usually described relatively concisely, such as "the patient is euphoric" or "the mood is predominantly sad with elements of frustration and anger." It is desirable to use the patient's own words, such as "the patient reports feeling 'scared to death'," or "she feels 'on top of the world'." Most moods can be described by using terms from six clusters or ranges, which we have chosen to call euthymic, dysphoric, euphoric, angry, anxious, and apathetic. Terms frequently used to describe moods in these six clusters are listed in Table 3–1. People with no psychopathology are likely to experience moods in each of these ranges at various times in their lives. A given mood may be normal or abnormal for that patient, but the MSE documents only the specific mood currently reported by the patient as observed by the examiner. Determinations of normalcy or pathology are incorporated into the formulation and differential diagnosis. Whether a given mood is ultimately judged as being abnormal depends not on the mood alone but also on related features, such as whether the mood seems congruous with the individual's circumstances and experiences, whether the affective intensity is unusually heightened or blunted, and whether there are associated signs or symptoms of a mood disorder, such as mania.

Patients whose mood is *euthymic* or in the normal range appear calm, consistent in emotional expression, comfortable, appropriately friendly, and reasonably cooperative. They may be appropriately concerned or anxious about their problems, but are not overly frightened or agitated. A normal mood is usually a sign of health. It may be diagnostically important if an apparently normal mood is incongruous to the situation or thought content, such as when a tragedy has just occurred or if the patient is highly delusional. Terms that may be helpful in describing moods in the normal range include calm, pleasant, friendly, euthymic, comfortable, and unremarkable.

Patients with a mood in the *dysphoric* range may describe feeling down, blue, sad, worthless, upset, hopeless, and frustrated. Commonly there are other symptoms associated with dysphoric mood (though they are recorded in the history or

Table 3.1. Six clusters of terms to describe types of mood and affect

Euthymic:	calm	Apathetic:	apathetic
	comfortable		bland
	euthymic		dull
	friendly		flat
	normal		
	pleasant		
	unremarkable		
		Dysphoric:	despondent
			distraught
			dysphoric
Angry:	angry		grieving
	bellicose		hopeless
	belligerent		lugubrious
	confrontational		overwhelmed
	frustrated		remorseful
	hostile		sad
	impatient		
	irascible		
	irate		
	irritable	Apprehensive:	anxious
	oppositional		apprehensive
	outraged		fearful
	sullen		frightened
			high-strung
			nervous
			overwhelmed
Euphoric:	cheerful		panicked
	ecstatic		tense
	elated		terrified
	euphoric		worried
	giddy		
	happy		
	jovial		

other places in the mental status report), such as difficulty experiencing pleasure even when engaging in formerly pleasurable activities (known as *anhedonia*), reduced concentration, insomnia, decreased appetite, loss of libido, feelings of remorse, and crying. Terms useful for describing moods in the dysphoric range include sad and dysphoric. Where applicable, more extreme or specific terms can be used, such as despondent, distraught, overwhelmed, hopeless, grieving, remorseful, and lugubrious. A mood in the dysphoric range is a hallmark of major depressive disorder (though these individuals can sometimes present as angry or apathetic), but also can occur in the context of a variety of other disorders including mixed bipolar states, schizophrenia, anxiety disorders, drug or alcohol abuse, medical disorders (particularly neurologic, oncologic, and endocrinologic disorders, and postsurgery and chronic illness states), and personality disorders. Pseudobulbar palsy (also called *emotional incontinence*) may look like dysphoria, but it is accompanied by significant emotional lability with frequent, brief episodes (often incongruent and inappropriate) of tearfulness. Moreover, sadness and grief are normal and expected in the face of significant loss or setback, and mild inexplicable transient sadness can and does happen to most normal people. Particular attention should be paid to suicidal indicators when the mood is in the depressed range (see Chapter 5).

Euphoria and happiness are normal moods when the situation warrants, but can also accompany some pathologic conditions. Though they may also present as irritable or angry, manic patients classically have elevated moods, often to the point of elation or giddiness. Rapid speech, impulsiveness, exaggerated self-confidence or self-regard, and hyperactivity usually accompany a manic patient's elevated mood. Abnormally elevated mood is not in itself diagnostically specific; for example, its causes include drug intoxication (marijuana, ethanol, amphetamines, nitrous oxide) and disorganized schizophrenia. Disorganized (or hebephrenic) schizophrenics appear to be in a silly mood because of unprovoked and inappropriate smiling and laughter. A rare form of complex partial seizure disorder known as gelastic epilepsy can also result in sustained, inappropriate laughter. Descriptive words for moods in the happy range, listed roughly in order of increasing intensity, include cheerful, happy, jovial, euphoric, elated, and ecstatic. Because they are often coincident with elevated mood in manic patients, poor judgment and grandiosity should be assiduously elicited when an elevated mood is present.

Anger is a common psychiatric presentation, especially in the emergency room setting. Other health practitioners frustrated in dealing with angry patients frequently turn to mental health specialists for consultation. Sometimes patients are first interviewed in situations where anger should be expected, such as after a confrontation with another caregiver, after a terrible personal loss, or after being taken into custody on an involuntary commitment. Anger is communicated in direct verbal statements as well as in indirect ways that should be recorded in other sections of the mental status report: hostile tone of voice, threatening postures, terseness, tense facial expression, glaring eyes, increased muscle tension, abrupt movements, violent action, and so on. Reflection on one's own life experience should suffice to remind most physicians as to what people look and act like when they are angry. Anger or the tendency to become angry with minimal provocation (*irritability*) is the most common alternate mood for manics who are not elated and is a frequent alternate mood for depressives who are not simply sad. Drug or alcohol intoxication commonly causes an angry mood, which often results in coming to psychiatric attention. Other physical conditions that can result in angry mood include complex partial epilepsy, head trauma, stroke, and dementia. Even more commonly, patients with neurologic disorders are irritable and affectively labile, especially when the prefrontal cortex or the amygdala is affected. Irritable demented patients may bite, hit, or kick caregivers. Psychotic patients are sometimes angry, especially if they are paranoid. Anger may occur as a predictable response to a delusion (e.g., if a patient suspects his wife of dallying with her boss), but also can happen as part of the psychotic derangement, without evident explanation (e.g., in excited catatonics). Poorly modulated anger is encountered frequently among personality-disordered patients, especially those in the narcissistic–antisocial–borderline spectrum. As examples, a patient with narcissistic personality disorder may lapse into rage and demand to see the manager if the customer ahead of him in the express checkout line is permitted to exceed the maximum number of groceries; a previously charming and flattering patient with antisocial personality disorder may become hostile and threatening when his or her demands are rejected or limits are set. In describing an angry mood, useful adjectives include angry, hostile, irritable, bellicose, belligerent, sullen, frustrated, impatient, irascible, confrontational, oppositional, testy, and outraged. It should go without saying that the observation of anger should prompt attention to the examiner's own safety and to the patient's increased risk of aggression toward self or others.

Mood in the *anxious* range encompasses fearful, tense, and apprehensive feelings and is a common experience in threatening situations. It may be accompanied by signs of autonomic arousal (so-called fright–flight–fight response). Anxiety occurs in normal individuals in danger or under stress (e.g., in soldiers facing combat, recently diagnosed victims of life-threatening medical conditions, parents of missing children, and students anticipating final exams). In terms of psychiatric illnesses, apprehensive or fearful mood is typical in the anxiety disorders (including panic disorder and phobic states). Anxiety also may signal the presence of paranoid delusions, atypical depression, neuroleptic-induced akathisia, dependent personality disorder, or organic states such as hyperthyroidism, drug intoxication (e.g., cocaine, amphetamines), respiratory compromise, or systemic infection. Nightmares are anxiety dreams occurring during sleep. Panic is an extreme form of anxiety described as an overwhelming and vague sense of imminent death or doom, generally accompanied by agitation and somatic manifestations, such as palpitations, hyperventilation, sweating, nausea, and perioral or peripheral paresthesia. In addition to panic disorder, complex partial epilepsy may produce paroxysmal episodes of fear and panic. During deep sleep, night terrors can cause awakening with a similar vague and overwhelming sense of panic and doom (not in the setting of a nightmare). Words useful for describing moods in the apprehensive range include tense, anxious, nervous, high-strung, worried, frightened, fearful, panicked, and overwhelmed.

A final category of commonly encountered moods is *apathy*, where there is no evident mood. Included in this category are severe states of denial or emotional shock in response to acute trauma or tragedy ("I feel numb"), some psychotic states (e.g., catatonia or very blunted schizophrenia), neurologic conditions that impede emotional expression (e.g., parkinsonism and prefrontal cortex disorders), and somatoform disorders (e.g., conversion disorder, where the lack of emotional response to an apparent physical impairment is called *la belle indifference*). In catatonia, emotional shock, and severe brain damage, emotional nonreactivity may be accompanied by even more striking findings such as muteness or physical immobility. In most of these conditions, the apathy or lack of evident mood is transient, lasting from minutes to weeks. Rarely, individuals have persistent and consistent impairment in the capacity for emotional expression and an impaired capacity to recognize any of their mood shifts that do occur; such individuals are called *alexithymic*. Alexithymic persons may be at greater risk for somatoform disorders, which involve the indirect expression of psychologic issues through somatic symptoms. Moods in this category can be described as apathetic, bland, dull, or flat.

Affect

Whereas mood is usually more of a sustained feeling state described by the patient, affect involves moment-to-moment changes in the emotional state and the external expression of these feelings as observed by the examiner. The patient's affective state consists of several components. These components are objectively observed and cannot be elicited by direct questioning; they should be monitored throughout the interview because they may change. In casual conversations that touch on a variety of topics, a normal person displays a variety of affects of varying intensities that are observable through behaviors like laughing, joking, smiling, frowning, or crying. However, affective expression can also be quite subtle. Affect can be conveyed by tone of voice, gesticulation, facial expression, animation, and posture. Often examiners can sense affect in nonspecific ways or by inference from their own feelings (see Chapter 1). For example, examiners may themselves feel sad while interviewing depressed patients, bored while with apathetic patients, or uneasy while with hostile or suspicious patients. Learning to attend to subtleties of affective expression is vital for psychotherapists and helpful in any interpersonal encounter. In fact, those who are inattentive to others' affects may be perceived as being unempathic and may even court danger by ignoring messages expressed emotionally rather than verbally.

Mood and affect may be described in the same phrase if they are concordant, such as "mood and affect are sad." However, in writing the MSE report, mood and affect are more often separately described, albeit in the same subsection. For example, a patient who describes him- or herself as depressed may have an affect that is bland and indifferent. On the other hand, a patient who denies feeling dysphoric may appear tearful and sad, thus having a depressed affect. When the emotional expression is at variance with the expected response to the situation or content of discussion, affect is described as being *incongruent* or *inappropriate*.

Affective expression is interesting in and of itself; it is the spontaneous depiction of a person's current emotional state, like a window allowing a glimpse into his or her mood. However, astute psychiatric examiners go beyond a mere cataloging of affects toward analyzing how and to what degree the affect changes. In this regard, affective expression can be thought of as varying in two dimensions: movement among the various possible emotions is called *range of affect*; variations ranging from a lack of emotional expression to extreme emotional expressiveness are described on a continuum from little to great *intensity of affect*. The rate of change of these two dimensions (intensity and range), known as *mobility of affect*, is also assessed; if affect is judged to change too quickly in either direction, the patient is considered to be labile. Affective change in response to external stimuli such as provocation by the examiner is a part of affective mobility, but can be more specifically referred to as *affective reactivity*.

In a written description of affect, objective comments on type (e.g., sad, angry, euphoric), range expressed, mobility, intensity, reactivity, and appropriateness are relevant. In general, notation of abnormalities is more important than notation of normal features. Descriptive phrases for affect type are similar to those that were previously listed for mood. For example, "Affect is anxious" or "The patient appears sad and frustrated." Terms used to describe types of affect are listed in Table 3–1, and terms used to describe the other parameters of affect are listed in Table 3–2.

Table 3.2. Terms to describe parameters of affect

Parameter of Affect	Normal	Abnormal
Appropriateness	Appropriate Congruent	Inappropriate Incongruent
Intensity	Normal	Blunted Exaggerated Flat Heightened Overly dramatic
Mobility	Mobile	Constricted Fixed Immobile Labile
Range	Full range	Restricted range
Reactivity	Reactive Responsive	Nonreactive Nonresponsive

The range of affect comprises the variety of types of affect that the patient is capable of expressing during the interview. Range can be full or restricted. A full range of affect means that a variety of normal emotions are noted during the interview; that is, the patient is capable of showing appropriate sadness, happiness, anger, laughter, seriousness, and so on, depending on the context.

It is pathologic, though not uncommon, for affect to be limited in range and/or to fail to respond to external stimuli. The term *restricted* describes an incomplete affective range. Patients with severe depression are characteristically sad and do not return social smiles or react to humorous statements; the MSE report would say that "Affect was restricted to the dysphoric range and is nonreactive." Range of affect is often abnormal in schizophrenia, affective disorders, prefrontal cortex disorders, and Parkinson's disease.

Changes in tone of voice, facial expression, body posture, and other forms of nonverbal communication offer clues about affect and are recorded under the appearance section of the MSE. For example, people may retain the ability to smile gently even when feeling distressed; or instead of shedding tears, the patient's eyes may very faintly mist. Even when subtle or evanescent, these affective expressions provide valuable clues about the true range of affect.

It is normal for the patient's affect to adjust in response to changes in the external environment and in the topic of conversation. This capacity of affect to adjust appropriately in response to external factors is known as *reactivity*. While a patient may have a full or only mildly impaired range of affect, he or she can simultaneously show inappropriate reactivity. If a patient fails to respond to normally evocative stimuli, affect is said to be *nonreactive*. Reactivity may be dulled in schizophrenia, retarded depression, psychic shock, or disorders that impair consciousness or self-expression.

The intensity of affect is evaluated in terms of the strength of affective expression during the interview. *Heightened affective intensity* is commonly seen in mania and in histrionic and borderline personality disorders. Histrionic patients are also melodramatic, seductive, and strikingly sentimental. *Blunted affect* reflects reduced intensity and is usually accompanied by reduced reactivity; it may be seen in schizophrenia, depression, or prefrontal cortex injury (see Chapter 2, abulia). More rarely, a patient with one of these conditions may completely lack affective expression or reactivity. This is known as a *flat affect*. When the clinician records "the patient has a flat affect" without further elaboration, this implies that there is no range, little intensity, no mobility, and inappropriateness of affect. Usually no special notation is made if the affective intensity is normal, but blunted affect is recorded if intensity is muted. Overly dramatic, heightened, exaggerated, or intensely expressive affect are recorded when the intensity seems too great. There are cultural differences regarding what is considered normal affective intensity.

The rate at which affect changes is the mobility of affect. A normal capacity to change is described as mobile affect, while excessively rapid and unprovoked changes indicate a labile affect. Extreme lability occurs in response to minimal or imperceptible stimuli, often incongruently (see below, inappropriate affect). *Lability of affect* can occur at different rates in various conditions. A brain-damaged (e.g., pseudobulbar palsy) or delirious patient's affect can be labile from minute to minute. It is not unusual for these patients abruptly to grimace, cry, or sob, only to return to a calm expression a few seconds later. A personality-disordered patient's affect can change over the course of minutes to hours. A cyclothymic patient's affect can fluctuate dramatically over a period of days. Inadequate mobility of affect is the opposite of lability and may be described in a variety of ways, such as being decreased or *constricted*. Even more extreme is a *fixed* or *immobile affect*, which denotes virtually no mobility of affect, manifested by an unvarying expression of one particular emotion. As described elsewhere, patients who exhibit no discernible affect whatsoever are described as *flat*, a term connoting both decreased mobility as well as lack of a specific type of affect.

Affect is normally appropriate to, or congruent with, the environment, topic of conversation, or situation. We expect laughter when a joke is told and sadness at a funeral. Affect is described as being inappropriate when the emotion expressed does not fit the situation or the topic of conversation. Inappropriate and incongruent affect are virtually synonymous terms. While the word *incongruent* offers the advantage of sounding somewhat less pejorative, *inappropriate* is conventionally used and also acceptable.

Inappropriate affect is common in psychotic patients, who may smile or laugh inappropriately as a response to internal stimuli like hallucinations or odd thoughts, rather than to the external environment. Often psychotic patients will calmly and blandly describe delusions of persecution, that should be terrifying, thus exhibiting incongruence of emotional and verbal expression. Because anyone may smile or frown occasionally in response to his or her own thoughts, inappropriateness should be judged in the context of the complete interview as well as how striking or intrusive the incongruence is. Manic patients laugh, are overly familiar, and make socially inappropriate jokes, but such behavior is often congruent with an elevated mood. This should be labeled as inappropriate affect only if it clearly does not fit the situation (e.g., joking and laughing at church).

It is usually wise to ask patients about any affective expression that is remarkable, surprising, or unexplained. For example, if a forlorn-appearing patient does not spontaneously discuss his or her emotional state, it would be reasonable for the examiner to ask, "You look very sad; is what we are discussing upsetting to you?" Moreover, mood and affect provide important diagnostic clues; examiners should allow their questioning and thinking to be influenced by the patient's affect. In the forlorn-appearing patient mentioned above, it would be important to probe for depression and/or suicidality.

Definitions

Affect The external manifestation of a patient's emotion or feeling state. Characterizations of affect are objective descriptions, whereas characterizations of mood are based on the patient's subjective descriptions. Mood is a more sustained feeling state, whereas affect should be more variable during the time spent interviewing the patient. Because affect is viewed as a dynamic or changing entity, it can be described in terms of intensity, range, and mobility.

Affective lability A state of increased affective mobility. Labile patients display repeated, abrupt, often dramatic, and usually unprovoked changes in the type of emotion expressed or in their emotional intensity. Lability is often an important indicator of neuropsychiatric pathology.

Agitation A restless, motorically hyperactive, uncomfortable state (see Chapter 2).

Alexithymia Patients who are alexithymic have deficient awareness of different mood states and diminished capacity to describe their feelings verbally. Spontaneous facial expression, especially of negative feelings, is inhibited. Alexithymia is thought to be common among patients with substance abuse disorders, posttraumatic stress disorders, and somatoform disorders. Similar deficits are sometimes observed in patients with autism, schizophrenia, or right hemispheric stroke.

Anxious mood An uncomfortable, tense, apprehensive, and vigilant emotional state. Anxious mood is not necessarily provoked by a realistic danger but generally occurs in response to psychologically perceived threats or danger. Anxious individuals are worried, tense, hypervigilant, sometimes psychomotorically agitated, often experience physical symptoms of overactivity of the autonomic nervous system (tremor, palpitations, nausea, sweating, enlarged pupils, rapid breathing), and have difficulty relaxing or accepting reassurance.

Apathy A mood typified by lack of interest and desire, accompanied by decreased reaction to internal or external stimuli. Apathetic individuals are poorly motivated, uninterested, and unemotional. Depression is a common cause of apathy. Prefrontal cortex dysfunction produces apathy, as seen in patients with structural damage, schizophrenia, and dementias involving this region. At times it is difficult to differentiate apathy from abulia (see Chapter 2).

Appropriate affect A normal state where the emotion apparent to the examiner corresponds to the content of speech and thought.

Blunted affect A state in which externally expressed emotion is present but much diminished in its intensity, as compared to what is normally expected. This contrasts with flattened affect (see below in this section) in which there is no emotional expression at all. Blunted affect is said to occur, for example, when a patient feels "numb" after a traumatic event and does not express the horror that he or she is expected to feel. However, blunting most frequently occurs in psychotic patients. A chronically psychotic individual may very blandly describe violent, paranoid thoughts. Blunted affect may also be seen in delirium, dementia, and lesions of frontal lobes or the right hemisphere.

Depressed mood   An emotional state consistent with sadness and dysphoria. Because of the association of the term *depression* with the diagnostic category, it is preferable to use less ambiguous descriptors such as sad, low, blue, down, or dysphoric.

Dysphoria   An unpleasant and negative mood that is perceived as being uncomfortable. While dysphoria includes a sense of feeling low or blue, it also has a broader meaning and includes a sense of malaise, discomfort, and uneasiness. This uneasiness is distinct from the tension and restlessness of anxiety.

Euphoria   Elevated, exceedingly happy mood, as if one had just fallen in love or won the lottery.

Euthymia   A normal mood that includes the expected little ups and downs of life, but not with the major or prolonged shifts of mood as seen in anxious, depressed, irritable, or manic mood states.

Fixed affect   The unvarying display of one particular affect or emotion throughout the interview, such as hostility or euphoria. Fixed affect implies absence of affective range and mobility.

Flat affect   A state in which there is no emotional expression. This is an extreme form of blunted affect (see above), in which there is essentially no emotional expression. The patient with flat affect also has minimal variability of facial expression, shows no gesticulations, and speaks in a monotone. This phrase indicates that there is no range, mobility, or intensity of affect.

Inappropriate affect   The emotion displayed does not match the speech, thought, or context accompanying it. The phrase *incongruent affect* is synonymous.

Intensity of affect   The strength of emotional expression. Passionate, excited people may be said to have intense or violent affect; in contrast, those with limited emotional expression may be said to have blunted or flattened affect. Normally, the intensity of affect is expected to vary according to the situation or with one's mood. There are also cultural and regional differences in what constitutes a normal intensity of affect.

La belle indifference   Lack of the normally expected concern for an apparently serious condition—for example, calm unconcern and acceptance in acutely paralyzed or mute patients. La belle indifference is associated with conversion disorder (previously known as hysteria) and various neurologic disorders. These patients typically lack insight regarding the emotions or conflict that underlie the conversion. La belle indifference should be differentiated from *anosognosia*, which is the extreme lack of awareness of a motor or sensory deficit, often a concomitant of right cerebral hemisphere damage. In its mildest form, when confronted with the disability, the patient admits it but is not appropriately concerned (*anosodiaphoria*). In more severe forms, the victim may claim that the disabled body part does not belong to him (see Chapter 7).

Mobility of affect   The ease and speed with which one moves from the expression of one type of feeling to another, and from one level of emotional intensity to another. People normally show gradual changes in both the type and intensity of emotional expression. These changes can sometimes be abrupt even in normal individuals if precipitated by external stimuli—for example, by very exciting or shocking news. The pathologic reduction of this normal emotional variability can be called *reduced* (or *decreased*) mobility of affect; alternately this may be referred to as *constricted* (or *constriction of*) affect. Extremely constricted affect in which the patient displays one emotion without variation is called *fixed* or *immobile* affect. If a patient displays no affect whatsoever, reporting flat affect should supersede any comment on affective mobility. In contrast to descriptors of decreased mobility, labile affect (or mood) refers to pathologically increased mobility of affect. Affective mobility is conceptually related to affective range and reactivity, which are defined below.

Mood   A person's predominant emotion or feeling state. Mood affects one's self-satisfaction, perception of the world, and behavior. People are generally aware of their mood, particularly when asked about it. Characterizations of mood are based on the patient's own description, in contrast to affect which is judged by the clinician's observation of the patient's feeling state and emotional expression. Many psychiatric physicians also view mood as a relatively sustained state, and term the changing and instantaneous feelings associated with ideas or experiences as affects.

Range of affect   The variety of emotional expressions that an individual communicates during an extended interaction. Normal individuals can express very different feeling states at different times, and their affects can range from sad to happy, from satisfied to angry, or from anxious to calm, and so on. The ability of a patient to express many different emotions, in appropriate contexts, is described as a full or broad range of affect. Those people who are limited to the expression of one class of emotions (e.g., the interrelated group of anxious, worried, frustrated, and irritable) are said to have a restricted range of affect. Those that display only one type of emotion throughout the interview may be said to have a fixed or immobile affect.

Reactivity of affect The extent to which affect changes in direct response to environmental stimuli. This is conceptually quite similar to mobility of affect, except that the latter subsumes spontaneous and internally driven affective changes as well as the externally provoked changes considered under reactivity. Patients who do not respond to provocative actions such as the examiner's joking can be described as having a nonreactive affect.

Restricted affect A limited or decreased range of affect. Though these individuals may have intense affective expression, they do not show many types of emotion; for example, they may seem incapable of feeling happy or comfortable.

References

American Psychiatric Association. *Diagnostic and Statistical Manual of Mental Disorders* (Third Edition-Revised), DSM-III-R. Washington, D.C.: American Psychiatric Press, 1987.

Campbell, R. J. *Psychiatric Dictionary*, 6th edition. New York: Oxford University Press, 1989.

Kaplan, H. I., and Sadock, B. J. *The Comprehensive Textbook of Psychiatry*, 5th edition. Baltimore: Williams and Wilkins, 1989.

Nicholi, A. M. (ed.). *The New Harvard Guide to Psychiatry*. Cambridge, Mass.: The Belknap Press of Harvard University Press, 1988.

4 | Speech and Language

Human communication occurs through verbal and nonverbal mechanisms. Nonverbal modalities include sign language, pictures, symbols, gestures, facial expressions, actions, and body positions. This chapter focuses on verbal communications, expressed through speech and language. Verbal communication involves letter symbols, words, phrases, and sentences, put together so that grammatical rules of structure, or syntax, will allow meaningful communications, or semantics, to occur.

There are both semantic and motoric (expressive) components to language. The *semantic* content of language refers to its ability to convey meaning. The *motoric* aspects of language include the proper articulation and assembly (according to rules of grammar) of the building blocks of words (phonemes and morphemes), facial and gestural (e.g., sign language) expressions, and writing. The left frontal lobe (see Figure 4–1) is particularly important for the motoric aspects of language, whereas the left temporal area is vital to the semantic aspects. The prefrontal cerebral cortex has also recently been hypothesized to play some role in semantic processing of language. As discussed further in this chapter, left frontal injury is associated with Broca's aphasia, and left temporal injury is associated with Wernicke's aphasia.

Over and above its grammatical, semantic, prosodic, and phonologic components, *pragmatics* is the aspect of language concerned with its overall communicative value. Whereas the dominant hemisphere (typically left) controls most aspects of language, the right side contributes to its communicative value. According to Cutting, the right hemisphere plays an important role in allowing a person to use metaphor and grasp the meaning of abstract verbal communications (see Abstraction and Conceptualization, in Chapter 6). This is an example of the right hemisphere's integrative functions, necessary to appreciating the "whole" picture and the implied meanings that underlie the overt content of communications (see Chapter 1, under The Interview as a Means To Elicit Information, content vs. process).

Although the capacity to use language is normally highly dependent on the anatomic development of specific cortical areas in the peri-Sylvian (around the Sylvian fissure, which separates the temporal lobe from the parietal and frontal lobes) region of the left hemisphere, language and speech are acquired abilities, not innately present at birth. As such, training is necessary, beginning with imitation and then education. This is usually accomplished early in life, beginning with babbling and utterances in infancy, single words by one and a half

Lateral surface of the left hemisphere

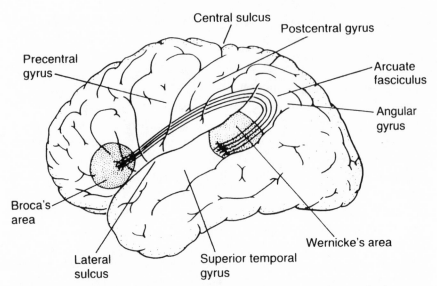

FIGURE 4–1   Diagram of the brain showing anatomic areas important for language. (Reprinted by permission of the publisher from *Principles of Neural Science, 3rd edition* edited by E. R. Kandel, Schwartz, J. H., and Jessell, T. M. Copyright 1991 by Elsevier Science Publishing Co., Inc.)

years, phrases by two years, and short sentences by three years of age. Damage to peri-Sylvian language areas (e.g., by stroke, trauma, seizures, tumor, or infection) produces various syndromes that involve the loss or deterioration of language and speech abilities. In addition, some conditions involve a developmental deficit of speech or language functions; these include the dyslexias and autism. Speech and language performance can be altered also by the presence of various psychiatric conditions, including mania, schizophrenia, delirium, dementia, Gilles de la Tourette's disease, and anxiety.

Language includes both the comprehension of word meanings, whether through hearing (auditory) or through reading (visual and vocal), and the ability to express them through writing or speaking. Whereas some utterances are probably more basic and perhaps associated with the evolutionarily older areas of the brain like the limbic system, sophisticated language and speech are largely human phenomena. Although unable to acquire formal syntactical language, some primates appear to be capable of learning some forms of symbolic and gestural communication, not unlike prelinguistic human infants. Nonhuman animals as well as preverbal humans may be capable of nonverbal thought. Indeed, thinking and language are not synonymous; logical and conceptual thought and perception can occur without language. In a similar vein, intelligence involves many abilities other than language and is likely present to some degree in nonhuman animals, such as dolphins, chimpanzees, and dogs.

Language function is highly lateralized, usually to the left hemisphere. Ninety-one percent of the population is right-handed. The left hemisphere is dominant for language in the vast majority of right-handers and in 60 percent of left-handers; however, left-handers also may have bilateral or right hemisphere dominance. It is important to consider the possibility of anomalous dominance when assessing atypical language problems. In addition, there are contributions to language from the right hemisphere, including that of pragmatics mentioned above, and a visuospatial aspect particularly important for the written expression of language.

Language deficits, known as *dysphasias* or *aphasias,* indicate dysfunction of the nervous system. However, aphasias can sometimes be mistakenly diagnosed as thought disorders (see Chapter 5) because both involve a disruption of the normal verbal expression of thought. There are important differences between aphasia and thought disorder, and in most cases careful observation and examination of the patient will discriminate between them.

The relationship between thought processes and language is unclear; thought occurs largely, but not exclusively, in a verbal medium. To some extent, spoken conversation reflects thought, in both content and structure. However, thinking and speech are not synonymous, nor are thought disorder and aphasia. Practically, it is very difficult to assess thought processes or to determine a patient's cognitive abilities when the expression or comprehension of language is not intact. Thus, to evaluate cognition (see Chapter 6), thought content, and thought process (see Chapter 5) in the MSE properly, one must first determine whether an aphasia is present and to what degree. Speech and language abnormalities or peculiarities may also be present as part of a constellation of signs and symptoms attributable to a particular psychiatric disorder even in the absence of a primary language disorder. Primary language deficits may be present concurrently with a psychiatric disorder; in these cases, the relative contribution of the psychiatric condition to the language abnormalities should be determined (e.g., a manic patient may have a stroke and become dysphasic). Conversely, aphasias are commonly associated with changes in mood and behavior; for example, Wernicke's aphasics may be euphoric and/or paranoid, whereas Broca's aphasics are frequently depressed.

This chapter contains information about speech and language useful for the purposes of defining primary language disorders as well as for describing the aberrancies that accompany various psychiatric disturbances. It is not meant to be an exhaustive review of speech and language function and terminology, but instead a general guide to issues important for psychiatric evaluation of patients. Unfortunately, this is often the section of the MSE to which psychiatrists pay the least attention. This may be in part due to the likelihood that dysphasic patients will be first seen and diagnosed by neurologists. However, with increasing numbers of neuropsychiatric patients being referred to psychiatrists, including those with head injury, stroke, or epilepsy, it is important to describe details of a speech and language assessment in the MSE. Familiarity with such details will enhance the examiner's ability to diagnose differentially and to distinguish the phenomenology of thought disorders, organic mental disorders, and aphasias.

Patients who are determined to have speech disorders that are not solely attributable to psychiatric pathology should be referred to a speech pathologist for more sophisticated assessment and rehabilitative therapy. Even if the psychiatrist proposes pharmacologic treatments with the intent to improve speech or language function, the speech pathologist can perform standardized tests to measure the patient's response to treatment.

Application

Fluency

Fluency refers to the initiation and flow of language, as heard in conversational speaking. There are fluent and nonfluent language disorders (see Table 4–1). In the most severe form of aphasia, called *global aphasia*, features of both the fluent and nonfluent types are combined and the patient may be noncommunicative.

Nonfluent language (and speech) means that the flow of language, whether expressed by speaking or by writing, is disrupted in some way rather than being smoothly initiated and executed. The most classic and extreme form of nonfluent language is seen in Broca's aphasia (see aphasias, below). Nonfluent language does not refer to lisps, dialects, injuries to the oropharynx, or other alterations of speech which are of motor (muscle-related) or peripheral origin.

Persons who chronically abuse alcohol or who have multiple sclerosis may have a type of nonfluent language dysfunction that is termed *scanning speech*. In fact, because of gait instability and speech defects, patients with multiple sclerosis are often mistakenly judged to be intoxicated. Appropriate words are chosen, but they are expressed in a halting fashion, with hesitation before initiating

Table 4.1. Disorders of language fluency

Nonfluent	Fluent
Broca's aphasia	Wernicke's aphasia
Transcortical motor aphasia	Conduction aphasia
Global aphasia	Transcortical sensory aphasia
Stuttering	
Cluttering	
Scanning speech	

phrases and inappropriate pauses. Nevertheless, once these patients have begun initiating the word or phrase, their spoken language is syntactically correct.

Stuttering is a common example, seen particularly in children, of a nonfluent deficit in the spontaneity and initiation of language. Stuttering involves multiple repetitions of letters and prolongations of pauses, and difficulty initiating phrases and words. An example is, "Are y-y-y-you go-go-go-go-going to the par-par-par-ty?" Letters or part-words may be repeated several times until the hesitation loosens and the flow continues. People are aware of their stuttering, so may become embarrassed or frustrated.

Cluttering is a more severe type of nonfluency than stuttering; it also occurs in children and can persist into adulthood. In cluttering, the prosody of the sentences is disrupted as phrases take on rhythms inappropriate to the grammar, thus altering the meaningfulness of the communication. There are abnormal bursts and pauses in phrasing, and rapid speech, resulting in severe cases in unintelligible communications. The clutterer is not aware of the language difficulty.

Aphasias

Aphasias are primary language disorders that produce errors in grammar and word choice. They are categorized broadly into two main types, fluent and nonfluent (see Table 4–2 and Figure 4–2). Many aphasias occur suddenly as a result of cortical (and sometimes subcortical, including thalamic) lesions such as stroke or tumor. There are individual differences in the deficits produced by a given lesion; some reports suggest that women may become less severely aphasic than men from an anatomically equivalent lesion. Intelligence, age, hemi-

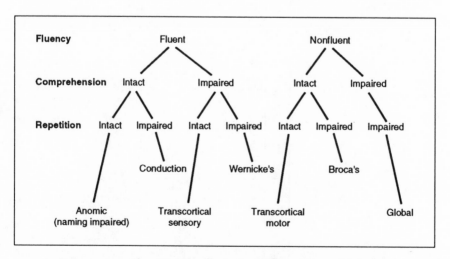

FIGURE 4–2   Flow Diagram Illustrating Differentiation of Aphasias.

Table 4.2. Characteristics of Types of Aphasias

Type	Speech	Comprehension	Repetition	Naming	Grammar	Prosody	Paraphasias	Semantics
Broca	nonfluent	normal	impaired	± impaired	impaired	impaired	some	meaningful
Wernicke	fluent	impaired	impaired	impaired	± intact	normal	yes	empty
Conduction	fluent	normal	impaired	impaired	± intact	normal	yes	meaningful
Global	nonfluent	impaired	impaired	impaired	impaired	impaired	yes	empty
Anomic	fluent	normal	normal	impaired	± intact	normal	yes	± meaning
Transcortical								
Motor	nonfluent	normal	normal	impaired	impaired	impaired	some	meaningful
Sensory	fluent	impaired	normal	impaired	± intact	normal	yes	empty

spheric dominance, education, and pathogenesis of the aphasia are also factors that may affect severity.

Nonfluent types

Persons with *Broca's aphasia* have *telegraphic* language—difficulty initiating words and phrases, abnormally long and misplaced pauses between words and phrases, and deleted connecting words (prepositions, conjunctions, articles) in their speech. Language is usually paraphasic (i.e., words or sounds are substituted for intended ones), and is effortful as the patient struggles to communicate effectively. Articulation is impaired, and the rhythm of speech is irregular. The result is disjointed communication. These abnormalities of speech can be detected in writing if the penmanship is legible. An example of language in a patient who has Broca's aphasia might be, "Thing went . . . door . . . he." Profane words can often be pronounced accurately, blurted when the patient becomes frustrated by the inability to express him- or herself. The ability to comprehend is usually relatively unaffected in Broca's aphasia, so the patient can follow instructions and is aware of his or her inability to communicate with others.

Transcortical motor aphasia resembles Broca's aphasia in every way except for intact repetition. The patient is able to repeat accurately something that is said even when he or she cannot spontaneously express it through speaking, confrontational naming, or writing. Reading aloud is impaired, although comprehension of spoken and written language is only mildly affected. The responsible lesion typically involves the dominant supplementary motor area and/or the white matter pathway connecting to Broca's area. In severe cases, this condition can be differentiated from mutism by asking the patient to repeat something that is said.

Fluent Types

The speech of fluent aphasic patients sounds flowing (*prosodic*) and syntactically correct, but there are significant abnormalities in the content and meaning of language (*semantics*). Unlike nonfluent aphasics, these patients speak in complete sentences. The classical example is *Wernicke's aphasia*, usually due to lesions restricted to the left temporal lobe, in which the patient has predominantly a comprehension deficit and produces nonsensical but well-articulated, prosodic language (*jargon*).

Paraphasias, the substitution of incorrect phonemes, words, or letters for appropriate choices, are common in fluent language disorders. There are two types of paraphasias: semantic and literal. *Semantic paraphasia* is the substitution of a correct word by another word in the same category, such as "cat" for "dog" or "clock" for "watch." *Literal paraphasia* is the placement or substitution of incorrect letter(s) is an otherwise correct word, such as "dunny" for "bunny."

Both types of paraphasias occur in Wernicke's aphasia. In Alzheimer's dementia, semantic paraphasias usually occur more frequently than literal ones. In psychotic patients, such paraphasic errors should be differentiated from neologisms (see Chapter 5); *neologisms* are entirely new, nonsensical words invented by the patient (e.g., "crumach"). However, some would classify neologisms as extremely severe paraphasias.

If one ignores the content and the meaning of specific words, the production of fluent aphasic speech sounds fluent because the grammar and syntax are largely intact. However, communication is jargonistic and meaningless. An example might be, "The man came to his boor and side by lamp in those warranties he toot. . . ." Patients are often unaware of the senselessness of their spoken or written communication and may glibly talk on and on. Unlike patients with Broca's aphasia, patients with Wernicke's have difficulty comprehending what the examiner is asking or stating. Patients who have significant Wernicke's aphasia are, therefore, likely to be incompetent to make important decisions.

Conduction aphasia is another type of fluent aphasia, most commonly caused by lesions in the arcuate fasciculus and related association fibers connecting Wernicke's area in the dominant temporal lobe to Broca's area in the inferior frontal convolution of the same hemisphere. Its chief symptom is inability to repeat spoken language, even though (unlike Wernicke's) comprehension is largely intact. Conversational speech is fluent with literal (phonemic) paraphasias and *anomia*. Confrontational naming is impaired. Patients are more aware of errors and may try to correct them. Writing is plagued by the same type of paraphasic errors that occur in spoken language. Reading aloud is impaired, though reading comprehension in silent reading is often good. The latter differentiates it from Wernicke's aphasia or dementia.

Transcortical sensory aphasia is an unusual type of fluent aphasia, similar to Wernicke's except that repetition is intact and speech may approach echolalia. Naming is impaired, as is comprehension. Transcortical sensory aphasia typically results from lesions that disconnect Wernicke's area from surrounding temporoparietal association cortices.

DIFFERENTIATING APHASIAS FROM PSYCHIATRIC DISORDERS
Aphasia and other primary disorders of speech and language need to be differentiated from language dysfunction or peculiarities that occur in psychiatric disorders such as schizophrenia, delirium, dementia, anxiety, mania, dyslexia, and autism. Language alterations resulting from psychiatric causes usually tend to be less severe than aphasias and are associated with other symptoms consistent with the particular diagnosis. In degenerative dementias, like Alzheimer's, the language defects tend to be insidious, progressing over a relatively long period of time. Schizophrenics or manics are most likely to have only temporary abnormalities of speech, which occur during acute episodes of illness. Even when

their speech abnormalities are more persistent, they tend to be associated with symptoms like delusions, hallucinations, and mood disturbance.

Frontal lobe dementias, such as Pick's disease, can lead to a nonfluent aphasia. In parietotemporal dementias (Alzheimer's), syntax and motor speech fluency are usually spared, but semantics and comprehension are not. Naming and word-finding difficulties are some of the earliest findings in Alzheimer's dementia, as semantic information is lost; semantic paraphasias are common. Early in Alzheimer's dementia, patients may be aware of their language impairment and try to correct themselves; thus such patients differ from many fluent aphasics. Demented patients may perseverate and even have *palilalia* (involuntary repetitions). Language impairment tends to resemble anomic aphasia in mild dementia; a transcortical sensory aphasia in moderate dementia; a Wernicke's aphasia in severe dementia; and a global aphasia in end-stage dementia. Diagnostic confusion may occur between later stages of Alzheimer's dementia and Wernicke's aphasia, but in the former there is likely to have been a preceding period of gradual deterioration. Also, language impairment in dementia is but one of a constellation of symptoms (wandering, memory loss, etc.), whereas it is the most prominent disturbance in aphasia.

In delirium, language deficits may be primary or related to cognitive deficits. Responses are often irrelevant and include paraphasic or articulation errors. Syntax and comprehension are also impaired. Writing is frequently impaired, and confrontational naming may be deficient. Delirious patients usually cannot pay attention to tasks and have concentration deficits that affect a broad range of cognitive tasks. On the other hand, aphasics can generally attend to tasks appropriately. Depending on the severity of delirium, delirious patients may perform better on confrontational naming tasks than do aphasics.

The loose associations of schizophrenia may resemble fluent aphasia. Neologisms and perseveration can occur in aphasia as well as in schizophrenia. *Word salad* (see Chapter 5), occurring very rarely in extremely psychotic patients, resembles severe fluent aphasia in its distorted grammar, incoherent speech, neologisms, and semantic paraphasias. Schizophrenic patients usually seem unaware of the incoherence or peculiarity of their communications; they may even switch between normal and deviant sentences in the course of a conversation. In particular, schizophrenics have loose associations; entire phrases or sentences jump from topic to topic without much of an obvious connection between the ideas, making their spoken language less communicative of meaning. The content of communication in schizophrenia is often bizarre. Schizophrenics may be overinvolved with the semantic and phonemic aspects of language: They produce peculiar words, rhyming, and neologisms and become preoccupied with different meanings of a given word. Paraphasias in schizophrenia may be of the semantic or literal type. While schizophrenics generally have intact comprehension, they tend to be concrete (see Chapters 5 and 6) in their responses. Word-finding difficulties and impaired confrontational naming are more common in aphasia than in schizophrenia. Unlike fluent aphasics, schizophrenics usually have intact repetition, naming, syntax, and writing ability as well as comprehension, except in the most severely psychotic cases. Schizophrenics are usually able to write to dictation, name objects, and, except in word salad, use syntax correctly (although, as schizophrenia progresses, syntax may deteriorate).

Word-Finding Difficulty

Word-finding difficulty (*anomia* or *dysnomia*) is seen in patients after closed head injury, Alzheimer's dementia, sleep deprivation, anxiety, delirium, encephalitis, brain tumors, and aphasias. Paraphasias and *circumlocutions* (talking around the intended word) occur in place of the appropriate words. When naming is deficient, it is useful to assess the patient's ability to recognize the identity of an object and its use or function (for *agnosia* and *apraxia*, see Chapter 6).

Nominal (or anomic) *aphasia* (see Table 4–2) is a type of fluent aphasia in which the patient cannot name things, either spontaneously in speaking or when confronted, but can repeat and has only mild impairment in comprehension. The patient is usually aware of this difficulty, unlike the patient with Wernicke's aphasia. Patients who have early dementia may be aware of their language and cognitive deficits, which they may try to conceal, although later in dementia there may be no insight into the deficits.

While anomia can be a component of different types of aphasias, it can also be an isolated phenomenon resulting from nonfocal causes, or occur in the context of behavioral conditions including delirium, dementia, severe anxiety, inattention, and sleep deprivation. Because anomia can occur in various brain-damaged patients, it is not diagnostic of a specific lesion or disease. However, recent reports suggest that damage localized to the left anterior temporal cortex can produce an isolated naming deficit without associated language impairment, which, depending on the precise area affected, differentially affects retrieval of proper nouns versus common nouns.

Prosody of Speech

Prosody refers to variations in the rate, rhythm, and stress in speech. It includes musicality, intonation, phrasing, and intervals. The right cerebral hemisphere seems to have a major role in the production of emotional prosody, whereas the left hemisphere processes variations in pitch and rhythm. Impairment of prosody can affect both expression of speech as well as comprehension of the meaning of another person's speech. Prosody adds an emotional dimension to conversation and can significantly alter meaning through the "process" (see Chapter 1). Aprosodic patients have difficulty expressing their own affective communications and interpreting others' affects (see Chapter 3, *alexithymia*). Anterior right-hemisphere lesions cause more expressive deficits in prosody, whereas posterior lesions cause more receptive deficits (analogous to the aphasia pattern with left hemisphere lesions).

Prosody may be affected in aphasia, as it is in Broca's aphasia, where rate and rhythm are affected. In Wernicke's aphasia, rhythm and emotional intonation, and hence prosody, are generally preserved. Patients suffering from dementia, right hemisphere lesions, and parkinsonism may also have defects in prosody. Regional differences in dialect can also affect prosody; for example, English spoken in the southern United States is more musical, and may sound more dramatic or expressive.

The *rate* of speech can vary from slow to rapid. Anxious patients may speak quickly, whereas depressed patients may speak more slowly. Those intoxicated with alcohol may become disinhibited and speak quickly and forcefully, often saying things they might not ordinarily. Speech is termed *pressured* when one is trying to squeeze in a lot of words in a given time period, such that others have difficulty interrupting. Pressured speech denotes a large amount of speech at a quicker pace, that is often, but not necessarily, accompanied by greater loudness and intensity. In manic patients, who tend to be loquacious and have racing thoughts, pressured speech can be accompanied by *flight of ideas* (see Chapter 5). In mania and severe anxiety, this urge (pressure) to speak occurs without a filter over whatever thoughts are occurring, and nearly all thought becomes verbalized, at the risk of adverse social consequences.

When there are long pauses between phrases or before beginning sentences, speech *latency* is said to be prolonged. Depressed patients often speak slowly, and sometimes softly, with longer than normal pauses between words, phrases, and sentences. Parkinsonian patients are slowed in a number of motor functions, including speaking rate. In patients with nonfluent language disorders, hesitations and difficulty initiating speech increase latency. Patients who are mentally retarded, severely demented, or intoxicated with drugs that suppress the central nervous system (e.g., barbiturates) may speak slowly. Autistics can have difficulty initiating speech and may exhibit *aprosodia*. Some people naturally speak slowly and deliberately.

The *rhythm* of words and phrases within sentences imparts different meanings, depending on where emphases are placed. Variations in rhythm or *cadence* also contribute to dialectical and regional differences in language (e.g., Cajun). In cluttering, the rhythmicity of phrases is disturbed, obfuscating the meaning of the sentences. Autistics have idiosyncratic stress and rhythm to their speech. Stutterers interrupt the normal rhythm of speech when they get "stuck" on certain words.

Intonation contributes to the musicality of speech. The pitch normally varies throughout a sentence, conveying emotions and imparting different meanings.

For example, sarcastically shifting the emphasis of "really" in, "You're really smart" demonstrates how intonation can alter meaning. Raising the pitch at the end of a sentence can turn it into a question. For example, "You are going to buy me a present" stated with higher pitch at the last word reduces the certainty of receiving a present. Speech in which the intonation and pitch do not vary is described as *monotonous*. This commonly occurs in depressed patients, who lack animation and have sparse interest or energy for socializing or pursuing pleasurable activities. Alexithymic patients (see Chapter 3) speak aprosodically, as do persons with parkinsonism and right frontal lobe lesions.

Quality of Speech

Quality of speech has several parameters, including amount, loudness, phonation, pitch, amount, articulation, and spontaneity.

LOUDNESS

Loudness of speech may offer relevant clues to the type of psychiatric or emotional disturbance. Particular words or phrases may be stated louder in order to increase emphasis or gain attention. Manic patients who are behaving without social sensitivity yell and raise their voices inappropriately, such as when telling jokes or making injudicious comments. Demented patients may scream uncontrollably, much to the consternation of caregivers such as nursing home staff. Persons who are delirious may also yell because they are confused or may mumble unintelligibly. Persons in pain may (appropriately) yell out. Psychotic patients in seclusion frequently yell out. Many persons raise the loudness of their voices when expressing anger or irritation. Hard-of-hearing patients often speak loudly, and people talking to them may also find themselves raising their voices. (Hearing-impaired patients often read lips, so in examining them it is preferable to face them and speak clearly; the examiner should also determine which ear is better.) Unfortunately, cognitive impairment and language barriers also tend to raise the voices of examiners.

Depressed patients may be soft-spoken, and suspicious persons may even whisper. Whispering in the absence of a laryngeal or related disorder may indicate conversion disorder. Persistent hoarseness may be related to vocal cord injury or dysfunction, recent intubation, influenza, or hypothyroidism. Straining or tremor in speech suggests possible motor dysfunction, including extrapyramidal disorders such as parkinsonism. *Vocal tics*, analogous to motor tics, are guttural sounds; alternatively, they may manifest themselves as nonlinguistic sounds (coughing, clearing the throat, squeaking, etc.) that occur repetitively and stereotypically in inappropriate contexts. Vocal tics often occur in Gilles de la Tourette's disease.

PITCH

Overall *pitch* varies according to age and sex. Pitch tends to be determined for a given adult unless voice training is undergone to alter it. Children and females tend to have higher-pitched voices than males, although there is overlap in male and female adult ranges. Men with relatively high-pitched speaking voices may surprisingly sing as basses. Pitch can vary during different mood states, such as in anger or agitation. Pitch variation also occurs in central nervous system disorders and disorders of peripheral anatomy. The variation of pitch that occurs in speaking phrases or sentences is called *intonation* (considered under Prosody, above).

AMOUNT

The *amount* of speech produced ranges from sparse to talkative. Loquacious persons may be manic, anxious, or attempting to control the interview. Wernicke's aphasia patients are often loquacious. Depressed persons may feel socially avoidant and speak very little. *Mutism* is the absence of speech and can result from psychiatric or neurologic causes. Mutism can be caused by a neurologic disorder such as a complex partial seizure or a mesial frontal infarction, or be due to a psychiatric disorder such as schizophrenia, other psychoses, delirium, autism, severe depression, catatonia, end-stage dementia, conversion disorder, and factitious disorder.

SPONTANEITY

Spontaneity of speech is the degree to which the patient initiates and engages in conversation. Depressed patients commonly demonstrate decreased spontaneity of speech, which is consistent with the associated paucity (amount), slow rate, impaired prosody, and reduced loudness. In contrast, manics are usually very eager to speak and do so loquaciously. Paranoid or suspicious patients may be hesitant to initiate conversation. Demented or delirious patients may have a reduced spontaneity of speech, in part related to their cognitive deficits.

ARTICULATION

Articulation is the pronunciation of sounds (*phonemes*) that comprise words. This includes vowels and consonants. *Dysarthria* may be due to either central nervous system or peripheral dysfunction. There are five types of dysarthria: spastic, flaccid, ataxic, hypokinetic, and hyperkinetic, depending on the underlying pathology.

Broca's aphasia patients may have articulation problems, especially if there is an associated paresis of facial and oropharyngeal muscles. Slurring of words may indicate intoxication from alcohol or motor dysfunction of the oral–pharyngeal area including the tongue. Chorea or tardive dyskinesia can alter articulation through abrupt interruptions of coordinated muscle activity, including that of the tongue and oropharynx. Drug side effects may impair articulation, such as dry mouth secondary to the use of anticholinergic drugs or sedation related to pain-relieving or sleep-inducing medications.

Dialect—the differences in speech that result from cultural or regional influences—can significantly impact articulation (i.e., pronunciation). In addition, dialects have their own rules for accents, prosody, and syntax. English is the common language of Great Britain, the United States, and Jamaica, but dialect varies significantly. Dialectical differences from standard American English can affect not only the intonation, rhythm, and choice of words, but also grammar, articulation, and phonology. For example, in some African-American dialects, final consonants are often deleted. Dialect is *not* indicative of speech dysfunction.

PHONATION

Resonance is the quality of speech contributed by the oral cavity in relation to the palate. Abnormality can contribute to dysarthria and reduce the intelligibility of speech. An example is hypernasality resulting from paralysis of the soft palate or cleft palate.

The Examination

Examination of language function should begin with a determination of the vision, hearing, and muscle strength and coordination status of the patient. It involves both direct testing of some skills and careful listening to and observation of others. It should include assessment of the following language functions:

1. Fluency of speech
2. Repetition
3. Comprehension
4. Naming
5. Writing
6. Reading
7. Prosody
8. Quality of speech

It is helpful first to know which side is the dominant hemisphere for language in a given individual. Tests may be needed to determine handedness. This may be accomplished at the bedside or in the office by having the patient perform a few tasks. Hand, foot, and eye preference can be readily assessed. The dominant hand can usually be determined by instructing the patient to write something. Occasionally, left handers are compelled during childhood to take up writing with the right hand, so dominance can be confirmed by requesting the patient to simulate other tasks such as striking a match, threading a needle, dealing cards, or brushing hair. Foot preference can be ascertained by asking the patient to simulate kicking a ball. Eye dominance can be determined by noting which eye the patient uses when instructed to peer through a half-inch hole in a piece of paper held at arm's length while focusing on the examiner's finger or a distant object. Then, the patient is told to close the left eye only, then open both eyes, then close the right eye only. The object "disappears" when the dominant eye is closed. The side of the brain that is opposite to the preferred hand, foot, or eye would be considered dominant in the majority of persons, except for some left-handed right-dominant persons. When laterality is not congruent for all tasks, the likelihood of determining language dominance correctly seems to be the highest with the writing test and lowest with the eye preference test. Many right-handed persons use their left eye to focus a camera, for example.

Special Situations

There are some special situations in which the assessment of speech and language (not to mention the other sections of the MSE) is difficult. Some patients may not speak English, or if they do, they may not be able to read or write in English. In such cases an interpreter is needed; at times, a family member can serve as the interpreter. Hospitals usually maintain a list of employees who speak foreign languages, and these individuals can be consulted to help in the patient evaluation. If capable, the interpreter may help in the evaluation of various parameters of language. Of course, in those instances, a reiteration about the confidentiality of the interview is necessary. Interestingly, multilingual patients who suffer from stroke, dementia, or delirium may revert to speaking their first-learned language, which may not be English.

Intubated patients are particularly challenging to interview. Using gestures and asking questions requiring only a yes or no response, which can be nonver-bally communicated with head-nodding, eye-blinking, or thumbs-up for yes and thumbs-down for no, can be helpful to elicit basic information and test basic comprehension. However, the examiner usually resorts to having the patient write down answers, a laborious process. In these instances a child's "magic" writing board (clear plastic writing sheet over special black cardboard) is more convenient than a notepad because it easily erases; on the other hand, paper is preferable if the examiner wants to document any language impairment evident in dysgraphia.

Patients who have had radical surgery of the head or neck (e.g., in treatment for cancer) may no longer have a vocal apparatus. Those who have undergone laryngectomy will not have a larynx (vocal cord box) and therefore are *aphonic*. A speech pathologist can be consulted to instruct the patient in the use of a portable speaking device, called an electrolarynx, which is held at the throat to amplify vibrations and sounds.

Deaf-mute patients usually can sign, although the interviewer will need an interpreter who knows sign language. Interestingly, sign language communications are also altered by the presence of aphasia. Blind patients may not be capable of writing neatly, and this should be taken into consideration in the interpretation of writing deficits.

Mutism describes a state in which the patient does not speak at all. Mute patients may be able to communicate using nonverbal means, depending on the etiology. In locked-in syndrome, the patient may be able to communicate using eye-blinking to indicate yes/no answers.

Although the dysphasic/aphasic patient has trouble with propositional speech, he or she is usually capable of *nonpropositional* (gestural or affective) *communications* and overlearned verbalizations. The latter include nonverbal utterances, especially those that convey affect, simple well-learned words like "hello," "no," and profanity, a familiar song, and overlearned material like the days of the week.

Fluency

Fluency is assessed by first carefully listening to the patient's *spontaneous speech*. Spontaneous speech can be evaluated by encouraging the patient with open-ended questions or by using a picture to stimulate conversation. Can the patient initiate and maintain a conversation? Is the speech telegraphic or monosyllabic, suggesting nonfluency? Are conjunctions and connectives omitted, such as "and," "to," "the," "but" (also suggesting nonfluency)? Do the words and phrases fall in expected places in sentences according to rules of grammar? Is there substantive content to the communication, or is it void of meaning? Are there prolonged latencies between words? (Latency should be less than three seconds in normals.) How many words are produced in a minute of spontaneous conversation? (Less than 50 suggests nonfluency, severe depression, catatonia, or mutism.) Normally 100 to 150 words per minute are expected. In fluent aphasia, increased output (e.g., over 200 words per minute) is common. Manic patients may also have increased verbal output. Reduced phrase length, often to single words, suggests nonfluency. Expletives instead of normal sentences suggest a nonfluent aphasia or Gilles de la Tourette's disease (or antisocial problems). Poor articulation (see below) may also be associated with nonfluent aphasia, as are frustration and effortfulness in speaking. Psychiatric causes include delirium, dementia, catatonia, significant mental retardation, autism, and severe psychosis.

Repetition

Repetition is assessed in the ability to repeat spoken words and phrases. Simple familiar words, such as "dog" and "school," should be tried first, then multi-syllabic words, such as "hospital." Next the patient is instructed to repeat short phrases such as "running into the garage," followed by simple sentences, such as "The spy fled to Greece" or "The postal service delivered the package to my neighbor." Finally, sentences with complex syntax are used, for example, "If the blue boat arrives very soon, we can go fishing for sharks." Conduction, Wernicke's, and Broca's aphasias impair even simple repetition. Patients who *perseverate* continue to repeat a task even after it is no longer requested. (Patients with schizophrenia, frontal dementias, transcortical aphasias, and autism may have *echolalia* that occurs during the interview at times when these patients are not requested to repeat the examiner's words.) Manics who are being sarcastic and uncooperative may also keep repeating just to annoy the examiner. Delirious persons may be unable to repeat long or complex phrases, because of their attentional deficits and confusion. Ability to repeat appropriately can help differentiate among the different types of aphasias (see Table 4–2 and Figure 4–2).

Some psychiatric patients will repeat their own words over and over inappropriately. In *verbigeration*, words, phrases, and even entire sentences are repeated (e.g., "going to school, going to school, going to school, going to school . . ."); these words were not previously part of a normal conversation, as in perseveration. Verbigeration is seen in schizophrenia and catatonia. *Palilalia* is also the repetition of one's own words, albeit at an increasingly rapid pace with progressively poorer articulation. Palilalia is rare and occurs in delirium, schizophrenia, Gilles de la Tourette's disease, aphasias, and basal ganglia disorders like parkinsonism.

Comprehension

Comprehension can be tested in both spoken and written propositional language. Adequate hearing should be established first, especially in the elderly. Comprehension should then be tested with a series of increasingly complex sets of commands. Because these commands generally have a motor component, impaired patients should be checked for apraxia or paresis.

Testing could begin with a simple single-step command such as "Point to your eyes," or "Are you wearing a ring?" or "Is it raining today?" Next would be a two-stage command—for example, "Touch your left hand to your right ear," or "Put the pencil under the paper." Then, a three-stage command of otherwise unrelated activities can be tried, for example: "Pick up the paper clip, put it on the table, and cross your arms." Comprehension may be intact for some verbally related tasks yet not for others. Comprehension is usually not completely deficient even in aphasia, although it may be in extreme cases such as delirium, severe dementia, and word deafness.

Comprehension may be intact for basic things or for concrete thinking, but not for more abstract thinking about complicated relationships and judgments. The presence of a significant psychiatric disorder, including dementia, psychosis, severe depression, severe anxiety, and delirium, can prevent full comprehension of subtle, abstract, or conceptual, words or phrases (e.g., peace, justice, truth, love). The examiner should test the ability to comprehend statements that involve comparisons and relational concepts, by using questions such as "If you buy an orange for 40 cents and give the store clerk a dollar, which coins do you receive in change?" Or "If Joe is taller than Richard and shorter than Harold, who is the tallest?" Patients can also be asked to read a paragraph from a newspaper or magazine article and then be quizzed on its content.

Naming

Naming of persons or objects is usually tested in the visual modality, but may also be tested in tactile or auditory modalities, which is particularly relevant for demented persons who have visuospatial deficits that interfere in visual confrontational naming tests. There are numerous ways to test naming abilities. A common approach, *confrontational naming*, is to point to a wristwatch and ask "What is this called?" and then ask the names of its smaller parts, such as the band, stem, and face. Sometimes patients can name whole objects but are unable to name the smaller parts. Alternatively, one could use line drawings from the Boston Naming Test (Kaplan, Goodglass, and Weintraub, 1983), see samples in Figure 4–3, to test naming; these drawings represent a range in difficulty from easy drawings like house or ladder to less common objects like abacus or unicorn.

If a patient cannot name an object (e.g., a camera), the examiner should give a semantic clue (e.g., "It is used to take photographs"). If the patient still cannot name it, a phonemic clue should be given (e.g., "The word begins with the sound *ka*"). If this does not help, a short list of words should be offered (multiple-choice) (e.g., "Which word is it—cabbage–school–microwave–camera–truck?"). More impaired patients require more clues, so it is useful to record how much cuing is needed.

A single scene with multiple details for the patient to point out and name may be useful (see Figure 4–4). The examiner requests, "Name everything you can see in this picture." Figure 4–4, the "Cookie Theft Picture," is taken from the Boston Diagnostic Aphasia Examination (Goodglass and Kaplan, 1987) and can be used to request names of persons and objects, as well as actions, such as

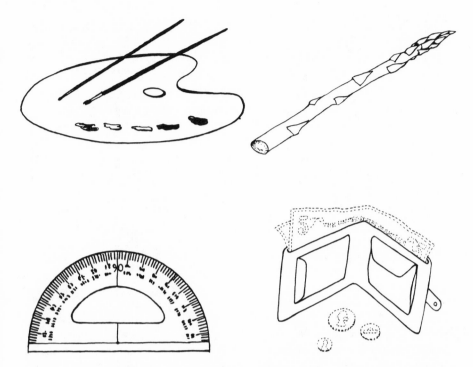

FIGURE 4–3   Sample drawings taken from the Boston Naming Test for use in testing naming ability. (Reproduced from E. Kaplan, H. Goodglass, and S. Weintraub: *Boston Naming Test*. Philadelphia, Lea & Febiger, 1983. Reprinted with permission.)

stealing from the cookie jar or washing dishes. This drawing can also be used to test other functions—for example, as a stimulus for spontaneous speech (see above).

Anomics, including closed head injury and dementia patients, also have difficulty generating lists of items from a particular category (e.g., wild animals, types of fruit, or things in a grocery store) or items beginning with a given letter (e.g., "things that start with a *b*"—boat, baby, banner, billboard, bank, etc.). Patients are usually instructed to generate as many words as possible in 60 seconds. Normals produce at least 20 words in a minute.

Alzheimer's patients may perseverate during word generation. Aphasics and patients with left prefrontal lesions are typically more impaired on letter than category fluency, whereas patients who are poorly motivated perform similarly on both. Bifrontal lesions produce severe deficiencies. Anomic patients may circumvent the intended word and purposefully retrieve a related word (but one that begins with a different letter or does not fit into the category); this would not be considered a true semantic paraphasia.

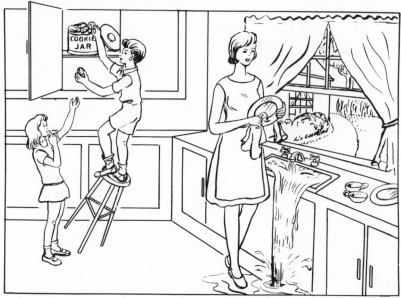

FIGURE 4–4   The Cookie Theft Picture, to test naming of objects and actions, taken from the Boston Diagnostic Aphasia Examination.(Reproduced from H. Goodglass and E. Kaplan: *The Assessment of Aphasia and Related Disorders.* Lea & Febiger, 1983. Reprinted with permission.)

Writing

Like speech, writing expresses language, so testing *writing ability* is another route to assessing language deficits. Usually writing problems mirror those in speech. Reading and writing can be impaired by a range of disorders, including aphasias, dyslexia, visuospatial deficits, and movement disorders (chorea, etc.).

After establishing that vision is intact, writing can be tested through spontaneous, dictated, and assigned narrative tasks. Although it may be practically useful to have the patient write his or her signature, this is so overlearned that it is too insensitive for use as a screening test of written language function. As in testing reading or repetition, it is best to begin with familiar things, such as writing a home address or months of the year. If visuospatial deficits are suspected (e.g., right hemisphere lesion), the examiner should have the patient copy some sentences and should check for perceptual distortions, such as the shapes of letters, difficulty with spatial positioning of lines in reference to margins, writing off the edge of the page, and so on. Next, the patient should write sentences of his or her choice for one minute. These sentences are checked for grammar, spelling, penmanship, semantics, and paraphasic errors. The sentences should contain subjects, verbs, and objects. Broca's aphasics write large

messy letters, misspell, and omit connecting words. Penmanship becomes especially poor when a paretic dominant hand is used or when the nondominant
hand is used. Wernicke's aphasics write more neatly than do Broca's, but use the
wrong words and have misspellings. Parkinsonian patients may write using progressively smaller letters (*micrographia*) as their disease advances. Interictal
temporal-lobe epileptics may write pages of detailed, idiosyncratic material (*hypergraphia*). Frontal lobe brain-damaged patients may perseveratively repeat certain letters (e.g., "mmmother" or "boook"). In these patients, letter substitutions
may be phonemic (e.g., *b* for *p*), whereas other letters may be deleted; entire
words may be incorrectly substituted (e.g., "tiger" for "house"), with words that
may or may not have any meaningful relationship to the correct word.

To seek more subtle deficits, the examiner can dictate several sentences, have
the patient copy sentences, or ask the patient to write a narrative summary about
a hobby or favorite activity.

Reading

Ability to read aloud and silently can be separately tested using sections of
newspaper or magazines, or other printed sentences. Print should be large
enough to be legible for elderly or other persons with vision impairment. The
level of difficulty of reading material should be adjusted based on the patient's
age and education. As the patient reads aloud, accuracy of words and sentences
should be evaluated. Comprehension is evaluated by asking the patient to describe what he or she just read.

The ability to read aloud does not necessarily indicate comprehension, but
does suggest an intact phonologic output system.

Unlike developmental inability to read (*dyslexia*), *acquired alexia* may be
associated with aphasia. Dyslexic children have difficulty reading, particularly
with comprehension, even though other aspects of their language are intact.
There are many different types of dyslexia, which correspond to particular
deficits, such as difficulty perceiving the shapes of letters, reversing letters,
and so on.

With aphasias, there may be similar defects in reading aloud as in speaking.
However, reading aloud may be dissociated from silent reading with comprehension. A patient with Broca's aphasia or transcortical motor aphasia may not be
able to read aloud, yet can often comprehend written material read silently. In
contrast, in Alzheimer's dementia reading aloud may be less impaired than
reading comprehension, because phonology and syntax usually remain intact
relatively longer than other aspects of language. In *alexia without agraphia*,
reading difficulties are dissociated from writing difficulties, usually as a result of a
lesion of the posterior corpus callosum and left occipital lobe. Such patients can
write meaningfully (spontaneously or to dictation), but are unable to read even

their own productions. *Alexia with agraphia* is due to a lesion in the left angular gyrus of the inferior parietal lobe.

Prosody

Prosody is assessed in the musicality and intonation of words and phrases and in the relationship of the intonations to the meaning of sentences. Monotonous speech is a clue to right hemisphere dysfunction, depression, or alexithymia. The overall rate of speech and variations in rate relating to specific topics of conversation may indicate anxiety or issues difficult for the patient. Pressured speech should be noted, as well as increased response latency, which occurs in depression and parkinsonism. Unusual rhythms or cadences are suggestive of cluttering or other nonfluencies. Because lesions of the right frontal and parietal lobes can alter the affective prosody of speech, other neurologic functions of these areas may need to be evaluated.

Quality of Speech

The examination for quality of speech should begin with observation of the patient's facial appearance. Asymmetries of the cheeks or mouth at rest or with smiling might suggest unilateral paralysis of a facial nerve or a stroke. The protruded tongue should be in the midline and free of choreiform movements.

The condition of the teeth should be noted, as edentulousness contributes to dysarthria. Articulation is tested by having the patient repeat phrases that do not have the expected grammatical structure of subject-verb-object; for example, "No ifs, ands, or buts," or "Methodist Episcopal."

Respiratory rate and ease of breathing can affect phonation; the underlying reason for whispering may be that the patient tires easily rather than that he or she is depressed. Hoarseness may be a clue to distinguish aphonia from mutism.

Other important quality of speech features to observe are pitch and loudness. Loquacity or its opposite, paucity of speech or even mutism, should be noted.

Definitions

Agrammatism   The inability to string words together in phrases or sentences using the rules of grammar. It may occur in speech and writing. The meaning of a collection of words is determined by their relative position in sentences as well as by the meanings of each individual word. The proper sequencing of words in accord with grammatical rules is called *syntax*. Syntactical errors occur in Broca's aphasia. Agrammatical speech lacks small words that are important to grammar, such as pronouns and prepositions; consequently, it is sometimes described as *telegraphic*.

Agraphia   A loss of acquired ability to write language. If the impairment is incomplete, it is termed *dysgraphia*. Because writing is a complex activity, it may be related to a number of cerebral functions, including intelligence, ability to comprehend written words, praxis, motor function, and visuospatial ability. Impairment in writing can occur independently of impairment in reading. It may also be part of an aphasia constellation. (See Dysgraphia in this section.)

Alexia   The loss or impairment of the ability to read. Comprehension of reading requires not only pronunciation of words but also understanding of the meaning of the written words (*semantics*). In alexia, comprehension of written language is impaired. When it is accompanied by an impairment of writing (agraphia), it is usually part of an aphasia. Alexia without agraphia is often the result of a visual–verbal disconnection syndrome.

Amusia   A defect in the appreciation or expression of music. Can be associated with Broca's or Wernicke's aphasia, or it may be an isolated phenomenon. However, some aphasics can use musical tunes to help retrieve words.

Anomia   Difficulty finding words to label persons or things, or difficulty naming objects when shown them, even though they are recognized as being familiar. Anomia is a symptom limited to word-finding difficulty; it can be present as part of an aphasia or other disorders, such as Alzheimer's dementia, increased intracranial pressure, delirium, conversion disorder, and other nonfocal brain disorders. The anomias of anterior aphasias, like Broca's, are the word-production type (phonemic), whereas those of posterior aphasias, like Wernicke's, are the semantic type. Anomias can also be specific to certain categories of things, such as colors or sounds. Mild anomia that responds to phonemic cueing may be seen in depression, parkinsonism, delirium, and normal-pressure hydrocephalus. Anomia involves a disruption of pathways between the language areas and the particular primary sensory areas.

Anomic aphasia   Inability to name objects and people despite relatively intact speech (except for some paraphasic errors), comprehension, and repetition. Writing is similarly impaired. Anomic patients are not apraxic and can demonstrate how to use objects. Anomic aphasia (also called nominal aphasia) is a type of fluent aphasia, with comprehension possibly only slightly impaired, confrontational naming (i.e., asking the patient to name certain objects on demand) defective, and repetition intact. It is often caused by lesions in the dominant temporoparietal area, but may result from lesions almost anywhere in the left hemisphere or from diffuse brain damage.

Aphasia   A loss or deterioration of the ability to comprehend and express ideas through language, including writing, reading, speaking, and comprehension. Aphasia is a central nervous system disorder and is not due to lesions of the vocal apparatus. The severity of aphasia can vary, ranging from mild word-finding difficulties to complete loss of expressive and comprehensive abilities. There are fluent and nonfluent aphasias, and *global aphasias* which are a combination of these types. Anomic aphasia involves a relatively selective loss in the ability to name aspects of people and objects. Insight into the aphasia varies with the type of aphasia; for example, Wernicke's patients do not realize the nonsensical nature of their communications, whereas Broca's patients are frustrated by their disability. Even when expressive language is very impaired, aphasics can still produce utterances that express some emotions. Simple well-learned words may still be intact (hello, yes, no, please), and, if the patient is disinhibited, profanity may be exclaimed. During fits of deep emotion, entire phrases may be suddenly and accurately expressed by aphasic individuals, as though impaired circuits have been bypassed. Cerebrovascular accidents (strokes), tumor, brain surgery, infection, and severe head trauma are causes of aphasia. The inability to acquire language in the context of global intellectual impairment, such as mental retardation, is not considered aphasia. Language impairment seen in schizophrenia, delirium, and dementia needs to be differentiated from aphasia. (See Fluent aphasia and Nonfluent aphasia in this section.)

Aprosodia   The loss of prosodic speech (see Prosody in this section). It is often accompanied by a decrease in gesturing. Aprosodia should be differentiated from alexithymia (see Chapter 3), in which there is a lack of variation and capacity for recognition of one's various emotional states. Some patients with right hemisphere lesions may be both alexithymic and aprosodic.

Articulation   The ability to pronounce *phonemes*, the smallest units of speech that are comprised of vowels and consonants, clearly and distinctly. Vocal activity is shaped by the action of the muscles of speech, including the lips, tongue, palate, and cheeks. Impaired ability to articulate is termed *dysarthria*. Normally each of these anatomic areas needs to be functional and coordinated in order to produce the different sounds of speech. Labial sounds are *b, p, m, w, u,* and *o.* Lingual sounds are *l, d, n, s, t, x,* and *z.* Palatal sounds are *b, d, m, n, g,* and *k.* Any disorder that affects oropharyngeal musculature, such as paralysis, stroke, multiple sclerosis, Bell's palsy, dystrophies, Friedreich's ataxia, and extrapyramidal disorders, may alter articulation.

Cluttering   A nonfluent speech abnormality that is jerky and rapid, using phrasing patterns that do not relate to grammar; there are inappropriate pauses and bursts of words. Speech can be unintelligible and is often rapidly paced. This pattern usually begins in childhood and may persist into adulthood.

Conduction aphasia   A type of fluent aphasia caused by lesions of the association fibers connecting Broca's and Wernicke's areas (including the arcuate fasciculus). In this condition, there are many paraphasic errors and impairment of confrontational naming, reflected in both spoken and written language. In particular, there is an inability to repeat words and to read aloud; however, comprehension is intact.

Coprolalia Compulsive and explosive profanity or obscenities. It is most commonly seen in patients who have Gilles de la Tourette's disease, but it is also seen in schizophrenia.

Dysarthria Speech that is poorly articulated because of damage to or dysfunction of the anatomically peripheral apparatus used to form words and sounds—namely, the tongue, mouth, palate, lips, throat, and muscles of the face. These muscles may be weak or poorly coordinated. Speech may be slurred or certain consonants may be enunciated improperly so that the spoken words are not easily understood. For example, the letter *b* may be substituted for the letter *p*. Errors of articulation include distortions, omissions, substitutions, and additions. Dysarthria should be differentiated from aphasia or dysphasia. It is possible to have a combination of aphasia and dysarthria in Broca's aphasia, if the muscles of the oropharynx are also directly affected, as is the case in a stroke in a large area of the dominant frontal lobe. Subcortical lesions, as in parkinsonism and brainstem strokes, and peripheral damage to nerves or muscles can cause dysarthria. In children, a host of congenital disorders that affect the development of the peripheral speech anatomy can cause dysarthria.

Dysgraphia An impairment in the ability to produce written language. This can be the result of a motor (*praxis*) defect or a linguistic defect. Motor defects are evidenced by poor-quality handwriting or visual–spatial abnormalities (such as letters and words not arranged correctly on the page or running off the edge of the page), substitutions of similar letters (*b* for *p*), or perseveration of the same letter. Deficits typically parallel the deficits in speech, including word-retrieval errors, paraphasias, and agrammatism.

Dyslexia A defect in acquired abilities related to written language, including reading, writing, and spelling. This term is applied to many different problems. Most persons with developmental dyslexia have normal intelligence, can comprehend language, and have intact primary motor and sensory systems. Many dyslexic children have deficits in visual or verbal memory. Those with visually related dyslexia seem to have a perceptual defect in that they cannot recognize shapes of letters, miss entire sections of sentences, transpose letters, or have difficulty scanning from left to right. Those with verbally mediated dyslexia cannot read aloud, and also make paraphasic errors. Dyslexia is usually a developmental learning disability and is often genetic. Dyslexia may also be acquired as part of an aphasic disturbance.

Dysphasia An incomplete aphasia (see Aphasia in this section).

Echolalia   The inappropriate and parrotlike repetition of another person's spoken words. It occurs in severe schizophrenia, catatonia, transcortical aphasia, and some dementias.

Fluent aphasia   The most common type is called Wernicke's aphasia (receptive aphasia), in which the comprehension of language is lost or impaired. The prosody and grammatical structure of speech is apparent; the cadence and rhythm of speech sound normal to the listener, and syntax is usually correct, but the communication is devoid of meaning. Expression contains word retrieval gaps and many paraphasias, and lacks semantic content (meaning). The speech rambles and wanders, often in a pressured fashion (*logorrhea*). Patients do not monitor their own performance and do not recognize their abnormalities. *Neologisms*, or made-up words, are also expressed. Intensely paraphasic and neologistic speech is sometimes called *jargon aphasia*. (Note that neologisms also occur in schizophrenic speech.) Writing is affected similarly to speech, with many paraphasic errors. The other types of fluent aphasias are transcortical sensory, conduction, and anomic. Transcortical sensory aphasia resembles Wernicke's aphasia, except that in the former, repetition is relatively spared.

Hypergraphia   A tendency to write excessively. This drive to write is seen classically in patients who have temporal lobe epilepsy; these patients write idiosyncratically on special topics and in great detail. It has been suggested that Dostoyevsky's writing was affected, not necessarily adversely, by his epilepsy. Schizophrenics and manics may also be hypergraphic.

Mutism   The lack of verbal communication. This may occur as elective mutism (in children, the refusal to speak even though language is intact), and in some deaf persons, as well as in catatonia, conversion disorder, locked-in syndrome, and end-stage dementias (notably the primary degenerative types such as Alzheimer's and Pick's). Large left mesial frontal infarctions involving the supplementary motor area may also produce mutism.

Nonfluent aphasia   The most common type is Broca's aphasia (motor aphasia), in which the expression of language is predominantly impaired while functional comprehension is mostly intact. (Broca's aphasics are impaired in tests of syntactic comprehension.) Fluency of expressed language is severely reduced, and grammar (syntax) is significantly impaired. There is relative preservation of the ability to speak automatized, well-learned sequences of words, such as the months of the year. Expletives may also be produced easily. Speech is somewhat dysarthric, lacks prepositions, adjectives, and connectives (i.e., is "telegraphic"), and is often monosyllabic, with poorly controlled loudness and little intonation. It requires great effort to initiate conversation, and patients are easily frustrated by their disability. Writing is similarly affected, with misspellings and omitted words (especially connecting words). However, the ability to copy written material is intact. The brain lesion associated with Broca's aphasia is located anteriorly, in the third convolution of the frontal lobe of the language-dominant hemisphere (the left side in most persons). Paralysis or weakness of limbs may be concurrent, depending on the extent of the frontal lobe lesion. Thus, writing must often be tested using the nondominant (usually left) hand. Other nonfluent aphasias include global aphasia and transcortical motor aphasia. The latter is distinguished from Broca's by preservation of repetition.

Palilalia The involuntary repetition of one's own words, parts of words, or phrases. Each word is repeated with progressively more rapidity and poorer articulation. It is rare, but is seen in Gilles de la Tourette's disease, pseudobulbar palsy, encephalitis, frontal dementias, schizophrenia, basal ganglia disorders such as parkinsonism, and transcortical aphasias.

Paraphasia The substitution of a letter or word for an intended letter or word. Paraphasias can be literal (phonemic) or semantic. In the semantic type, the substitution is of a word that is semantically related ("wife" for "mother," "clock-band" for "wristwatch"). In the literal (phonemic) type, an unintended substitution of a sound or syllable occurs (*m* for *b*, "moat" for "boat"), despite proper articulation. Paraphasias occur in conduction, anomic, Broca's, and Wernicke's aphasias, as well as in dementias, delirium, sleep deprivation, and other disorders involving word-finding difficulty.

Phonation The production of speech due to vocal cord vibrations and activity of the respiratory and laryngeal muscles; these determine loudness, quality, and pitch of spoken language. The flow of air past the vocal cords forms the sounds of spoken language. When impaired, speech is well articulated but whispered (laryngeal cancer), hoarseness may be present (nodules on the vocal cords), or the pitch is altered (with the flu). *Aphonia*, the loss of voice, is caused not by a cortical lesion but, rather, by a peripheral problem, such as that involving the vocal cords or the ability to breathe effectively.

Pragmatics The communicative value of language beyond the meaning derived from syntax, prosody, phonology, and semantics. The right hemisphere plays a major role in allowing the individual to appreciate these more abstract levels of language communication.

Pressured speech Speech that is particularly "driven" in amount, rate, and, often, loudness, as though the patient is compelled (pressured) to produce large amounts of speech in a short time. It occurs to some extent in persons who are very anxious, in those under great stress, and occasionally in hyperthyroidism. In its most classic form, pressured speech is associated with mania, or with disorders that include manic symptoms such as schizoaffective disorder or mood disorders secondary to medical illnesses or central nervous system disease. It may be accompanied by flight of ideas (see Chapter 5).

Prosody The qualities of speech that relate to rate, rhythm, amount, and intonation. Prosody, along with grammar and semantics, contributes to the expression of meaning and affective tone of language. Even slight shifts in prosody can subtly alter the meaning of speech. One important aspect of prosody is the "musicality" of speech, which refers to the variations of stress and melodic contour that are modulated within a sentence in order to make speech expressive and emotive. Without this aspect of prosody, speech would sound monotonous and flat. An example of the importance of prosody is sarcasm, which can dramatically alter the meaning of a sentence, even though grammar and content are unchanged. The right (or nondominant) cerebral hemisphere plays a major role in prosody. This is in contrast to the role that the left (or dominant) hemisphere plays in propositional language functions.

Scanning speech Nonfluent speech that is slowed and deliberate, with irregular emphasis on syllables. It reflects cerebellar dysfunction, as in multiple sclerosis, after trauma, and in chronic alcoholism.

Semantics The content or meaning imparted by language. Sentences impart meaning in part through the words that comprise them but also through their varying grammatical structures (phrases, commas, etc.). For example, the meaning imparted by the following two sentences differs significantly because of syntactical differences: "Finally, serve the dessert." "The dessert was finally served." Compare also these two sentences: "The steak was well done." "The steak was done well."

Stuttering A motor speech disorder characterized by the involuntary repetition of beginnings of words or phrases (including part-words), inappropriate prolongations of sounds or syllables, and abrupt halting. It is a disturbance of the normal fluency and timing of speech. It is a relatively common disorder that has various etiologies, including developmental deficit (most common), stroke, head injury, and psychologic abnormalities. Anxiety frequently worsens stuttering.

Syntax The rules of grammar, sentence structure and formation, and word usage that define the internal structure of language, including the sequence and hierarchy in which the components of a sentence appear. Words are arranged in an orderly sequence so that clauses, phrases, and sentences communicate meaning and ideas. Syntax is altered in Broca's aphasia and end-stage dementia.

Tic, vocal type A sudden, brief, unexpected, stereotyped, repetitive, and involuntary vocalization of a nonlinguistic sound. It includes coughing, grunting, snorting, and a variety of guttural sounds. When words are uttered, the tic is considered a verbal type. It is common in Gilles de la Tourette's disease (see Chapter 2).

Verbigeration   The incessant repetition of words, phrases, or sentences, generally inappropriate to the context or conversation. It is seen in schizophrenia and in catatonic states. It can be distinguished from perseveration in which words initially appropriate in a conversation are later repeated inappropriately.

Word deafness   An inability to comprehend anything spoken, although speaking, reading, and hearing are intact. It is usually due to a lesion in the left temporal lobe or to bilateral superior temporal lobe lesions. It must be differentiated from Wernicke's aphasia and deafness.

Word-finding difficulty   Inability to recall words or names of things spontaneously when engaged in conversation or during confrontational naming (when the patient is asked to name objects, body parts, etc.). It is seen in patients suffering from aphasia, dementia, brain damage, anxiety, and sleep deprivation.

Word salad   A term applied to extremely psychotic patients whose communications are incomprehensible and incoherent, as their words do not relate to each other in any meaningful way and may not be in proper syntactical relationships. Word salad may be difficult to distinguish from fluent aphasia (see Chapter 5).

References

Benson, D. F. *Aphasia, Alexia, and Agraphia*. New York: Churchill Livingstone, 1979.

Butterworth, G., and Grover, L. The origins of referential communication in human infancy. In *Thought Without Language*, ed. L. Weiskrantz. Oxford: Clarendon Press, 1989, Chapter 1, pp. 5–24.

Critchley, E.M.R. *Language and Speech Disorders*, London: CNS Publishers, 1987.

Cutting, J. *The Right Hemisphere and Psychiatric Disorders*. New York: Oxford University Press, 1990.

Damasio, A. R. Aphasia. *New England Journal of Medicine* 326: 531–539, 1992.

Espir, M.L.E., and Rose, F. C. *The Basic Neurology of Speech and Language*. Boston: Blackwell Scientific Publications, 1983.

Goodglass, H., and Kaplan, E. *The Assessment of Aphasia and Related Disorders*, 2nd edition. Philadelphia: Lea & Febiger, 1987.

Kaplan, E. F., Goodglass, H., and Weintraub, A. *The Boston Naming Test*, 2nd edition. Philadelphia: Lea & Febiger, 1983.

5 | Thought Process, Thought Content, and Perception

Although we cannot directly know another person's thoughts, inferences can be made based on what is said and observed. Assuming that there is no gross brain damage, which would cause language deficits (see Aphasias, in Chapter 4), evaluation of thought content and processes is critical to evaluating a patient's psychiatric state. Serious disorders of thought content and process, also known as psychotic disorders, are among the most severe and most disabling of psychiatric illnesses.

A classic example of thought disorder is schizophrenia. Schizophrenic patients can display any of a variety of disorders of thinking, including delusions, hallucinations, loose associations, ideas of reference, and thought blocking.

While disorders of thought are usually associated with the schizophrenic disorders, they can also occur in a variety of conditions. Severe cases of mania often are associated with hallucinations, delusions (typically grandiose or persecutory in nature), and flight of ideas. Severe depression can be of a psychotic depth and accompanied by delusions (often persecutory, nihilistic, or somatic in nature) and hallucinations. Delirium and advanced dementia usually include delusions (often persecutory), hallucinations, and incoherence. Personality-disordered patients—in particular, those of the borderline type—often use immature defense mechanisms that are associated with psychosis, such as splitting, denial, and projection (see Chapter 7), and may at times slip into overtly psychotic symptoms, such as hallucinations or delusions. Some drug intoxication and withdrawal states include thought disorder and psychosis; phencyclidine or meperidine intoxication and alcohol withdrawal delirium are examples of these.

A sense of what psychotic thinking is like may be gained by reflection on the thought processes of the dream state or of early childhood. Early in human development, thinking is *primary process*, similar to the strange and illogical thought processes of dreams and nightmares. Young children experience primary process thinking, for example, when they cannot differentiate fantasied monsters from reality, or when they engage in a great deal of magical thinking. In parallel with the development of the brain and personality through early life, secondary-process thinking evolves. *Secondary process* thought is the normal thinking process of the healthy, awake, alert human; it requires the ability to distinguish reality from fantasy and self from others, as well as the capacity for logical thought process.

Thinking appears to be both verbal and nonverbal in nature. Many adults think in words, although at a much faster pace than when speaking. Adults, and likely also children and infants, think in images as well. Interestingly, deaf-mute persons who have a thought disorder, such as schizophrenia, reveal abnormal thinking in their sign language. Thus, while intact language makes it easier to communicate with a patient and diagnose a thought disorder, thinking is a process that involves more than language; disruptions of thought usually occur independently of disruption of language, and vice versa.

Thinking has not been well-localized to any particular anatomic area in the brain, and may be subserved by many different regions, especially the association cortices. Thinking is difficult to study, since persons being studied need to have some language ability or symbolic communication to relate to others what they are thinking. Advanced brain-imaging techniques are beginning to localize the brain areas involved in analytical thinking, such as mathematical calculation. Overall, knowledge of the anatomy of thinking remains rudimentary.

The description of thought in this chapter is divided into process (flow and organization) and content. These are discussed separately, with particular attention to common abnormalities of thought, such as delusions, obsessions, phobias, and violent ideation. Hallucinations are also considered here, though they are more specifically a disturbance of perception than of thought per se. However, these complex nonverbal percepts may share similar neurologic substrates with thoughts.

Application

General Comments

Thought content and process are important parameters in the detection and documentation of psychosis. *Psychosis* is a general term that, in the broadest sense, refers to the dysjunction of thinking from reality. The most classic and undisputed symptoms of psychosis are delusions and hallucinations (abnormal thought content) and loosening of associations (abnormal thought process). Currently, clinicians often broaden psychosis to include abnormalities of appearance, affect, socialization, and volition. The terms *positive symptoms* and *negative symptoms* have been popularized by schizophrenia researchers and, therefore, are discussed largely in the context of that disorder. However, there is no fundamental reason to avoid these terms in describing other psychotic conditions. In broad terms, it is easiest to remember that a positive symptom is the "addition" of some attribute or behavior not normally present. Positive psychotic symptoms include delusions, hallucinations, ideas of reference, agitated and bizarre behavior, loose associations, neologisms, blocking, hostility, and affective lability. Analogously, negative symptoms can be thought of as a lack of attributes or abilities that are normally present. Negative psychotic symptoms include blunted or inappropriate affect, apathy, lack of motivation, social isolation, withdrawal, neglect of personal appearance, paucity of thought, and incapacity for abstraction.

The thought content and process portion of the MSE has great importance in the diagnosis of psychosis not only in schizophrenia, but also in other disorders, such as major depression, mania, or drug intoxication (e.g., amphetamines or PCP) or withdrawal (e.g., delirium tremens), and a variety of other neurologic or systemic derangements. Attention to thought content is important in understanding the patient's personality, situation, and chief complaint. Assessment of thought content is particularly vital in detecting dangerousness to self and others. Abnormalities of thought content are noted in a number of conditions. These themes will be elaborated below.

Thought Process

The goal of the examiner is to document an assessment of the patient's organization, flow, and production of thought. As the clinician cannot actually know patients' thoughts or thought processes, this assessment is inferred from patients' communication or from direct questioning about what their thoughts are like. Unless patients express their thoughts through speaking, writing, or sign language, their thought processes cannot be described. It is assumed that spoken words closely resemble the underlying thoughts. (Because disorders of thought process are typically expressed through speaking, some clinicians might record these abnormalities in the speech and language portion of the MSE. We prefer to describe evidence of primary language disturbance in the Speech and Language section, and evidence of thought process disturbance in this section of the MSE.) The presence of dysphasia or mutism makes determinations of thought processes much more difficult; however, aberrations of thought process may occur in both primary psychotic and secondary psychotic ("organic") disorders. Documentation of these aberrations is based on the examiner's observation of the patient's whole presentation, rather than solely on the patient's report of symptoms or responses to specific questions. As such, disorder of thought process may indicate psychopathology in a patient who is unwilling to acknowledge psychotic symptoms.

There is variation in the style of thought processes in normal people, both intra- and interindividually. The topics of speech and thought normally fluctuate as different ideas enter into consciousness. While these ideas may be more or less well-connected, depending on the circumstances, a person whose thoughts are always well organized and logical would probably be dull and uncreative. Thus, a determination that thought processes are "abnormal" is a judgment made by the examiner, based on the presence and frequency of specific phenomena.

Consequently, speech that a psychiatrist describes as loosely associated might in another context be considered poetry. Because disruptions of thought process are important indicators of psychopathology, these judgments should be made. However, in fairness to the patient and for accuracy of the examination, these judgments should be made as carefully as possible. Difficulties with inaccuracies can be minimized by basing conclusions on as much information as possible, and by including a description of the abnormality and its associated features, and an estimate of its severity, supported by specific examples in the MSE report.

Upon completion of the interview, the examiner should reflect on his or her overall impressions. Was the conversation direct and informative, or was it confusing and vague? Was it easy to gather information, or did the examiner have to work hard at asking questions to elicit information? Did the patient answer questions directly, or did questions need to be repeated and rephrased? Close attention should be paid to the patient's responses to open-ended questions or other opportunities to initiate or engage in conversation. Did the patient speak spontaneously, and what did he or she talk about? How smoothly did ideas flow one from another? Did the patient talk in circles, run on to different subjects, or switch topics abruptly? Were there specific examples of loose associations, blocking, or neologisms? Did the patient keep returning to one theme or perseveratively repeat the same words? Did the patient lapse into silence when not prompted by questions?

Under the thought process section of the MSE report, the organization (i.e., associations, connectedness) of thinking should be noted. Signs to include are peculiarities of thought processes, such as neologisms, blocking, clanging, circumstantiality, word salad, or perseveration (see Table 5–1). In describing the organization of speech, some clinicians make a global statement: "Thoughts are

Table 5.1. Important abnormalities of thought process

Disordered Connectedness and Organization of Thought

Circumstantiality
Flight of ideas
Loose associations
Tangentiality
Word salad

Other Peculiarities of Thought Process

Clang associations
Echolalia
Neologisms
Perseveration
Thought blocking

(mildly, moderately, severely) disorganized," or "Thoughts are rambling." Although this is acceptable, it is preferable to use more specific terms, such as "well-organized," "tangential," or "loose associations."

DISRUPTIONS OF CONNECTEDNESS

Circumstantiality and tangentiality are relatively mild forms of thought disorder; worse disruptions in increasing order of severity are flight of ideas, loose associations, word salad, and incoherence. Speech is organized into units of increasing size: Letters comprise words, words comprise phrases, phrases comprise sentences, and sentences comprise paragraphs that are normally structured in a proper syntactical organization (following rules of grammar). In thought disorders, the rules of syntax are generally preserved, although with loose associations, the logical flow of ideas in paragraphs is disrupted; sentences or even phrases may not be thematically connected to the preceding ones. In word salad, even the integrity of phrases is lost, and the words are no longer meaningfully connected to one another. Word salad is the form of thought disorder most difficult to distinguish from fluent aphasia.

Normal conversation (and by inference, the thinking underlying it) has organization. The topic changes at times, but in general, statements remain interrelated for at least a few sentences at a time. The connection of statements to those that precede or follow is generally clear, although an occasional odd connection is acceptable. When queried, persons without a thought disorder can logically reconstruct the series of (unexpressed) thoughts that had produced apparent shifts in topic. For the most part, questions are answered in a focused way without the need for redirection by the examiner.

Conversations with patients who exhibit *tangentiality* generally make sense and can be followed. On reflection, however, the interviewer realizes that the topic of conversation had strayed down another path or direction (tangent) without eventually returning to the original topic. For example, after starting out to answer a question as to who comprises her household, a patient may embark on a discourse regarding how she gets along with her sister. Some tangentiality is a feature of normal conversation, so describing a patient as tangential requires a judgment by the examiner that the digressions and tangents occur excessively. When interviewing tangential patients, the examiner must frequently redirect them back to the original or intended topic (i.e., a more "structured" interview style is frequently required). Tangential speech may be inefficient or time-consuming, but is not in itself conclusive evidence of psychosis.

Circumstantiality means "talking around" a topic. Such speech is digressive and overly detailed, but eventually returns to the original topic or makes the relevant point (if it fails to accomplish this, the speech should be described as circumstantial and tangential). For example, while explaining what led them to seek medical help, circumstantial patients may, before mentioning their chief complaint, detail their deliberations and various discussions with friends and relatives regarding the benefits and detriments of seeing a psychiatrist. Like tangentiality, this can be frustrating to the examiner, especially when under time constraints. The structure and productivity of interviews with circumstantial patients can be increased through directive questions and interruption of digressions. Circumstantiality is seen most commonly in obsessive patients, but can also be seen in psychosis and neurologic conditions, including mild delirium and temporal lobe epilepsy.

Flight of ideas is a thought disorder in which tangential associations occur quickly frequently (every one to two sentences or so); it is often concurrent in manic patients with pressured speech. For example, a patient might rapidly say:

I'm here because my mother sent me. She drove me in her car. The car is a Lincoln, and Lincoln is my favorite president. I don't know why they killed him. I've never thought of killing anybody because I love people, but only my dog loves me. Dogs have a terrible life, caged up and beaten all the time. People are caged up in prison. Could I go to prison for touching women? I like older women. I bought perfume for an old woman once. Perfume counters are so confusing. I heard that Bloomingdale's was sued for spraying perfume. There are too many lawyers.

Each sentence is more or less logically connected to the preceding one, but the topic repeatedly changes before elaboration of each thought can occur. This is seen most often in manics, typically in conjunction with pressured speech.

Episodes of almost complete disintegration of connectedness of subject matter in conversation and thought is referred to as *loosening of associations* (or loose associations). In flight of ideas there is still an obvious connectedness between the ideas and topics, but in loosening of associations there is no discernible topical connection between statements, or the apparent connection is not a logical one. The author was wearing a necktie with small whales imprinted on it while interviewing a schizophrenic patient. The patient spontaneously commented: "There are whales on your tie. My body is filled with sperm. Sperm is spilling out of me." One might conclude that the patient was connecting these ideas because of his knowledge of "sperm whales," but this is neither logical nor explicit, and would be referred to as a loose association (as well as a somatic delusion, if he really believed that sperm was spilling from him). If he were displaying flight of ideas instead, the patient might have rapidly said: "There are whales on your tie. I know something about whales because I read Melville's *Moby Dick*. How could he write such a long book? Moby Dick was a sperm whale. They call him that because he is shaped like sperm. I think sperm are disgusting. They can swim upstream. I like to swim." This could also be labeled as tangential speech; however, the degree of abruptness and repetitiveness of shifting topics is more severe, justifying the designation as flight of ideas.

Loosening of associations occurs to some degree in the majority of acutely psychotic patients and may be the only evidence of psychosis in patients who are adequately self-controlled and insightful to conceal their hallucinations and delusions. The severity of the loosening may be reduced as the examiner structures the interview; the responses tend to be more focused when the questions are more directive and less open-ended. Conversely, an interviewer may purposely avoid structuring in an effort to enhance detection of disordered thinking. The patient's writing will exhibit the same looseness of associations (see Figure 5–1); however, such patients can usually read aloud or copy from written material without difficulty, and some may even be able to sing verses in a more connected manner than they could speak them. This demonstrates that thought disorder primarily affects thought rather than language (see Aphasias, in Chapter 4).

Healthy individuals may at times display apparent loosening of associations: for example, when they follow a train of thought without vocalizing the intermediate steps, or when they abruptly change the topic. Unlike the psychotic patient, healthy individuals are able to detail lucidly the hidden series of thoughts that preceded the jumps in their overt (spoken) train of thought.

The presence of loose associations usually indicates a thought disorder and psychosis. They are most often associated with schizophrenia, and were a cornerstone to the Bleulerian approach to diagnosing this illness (this diagnostic system has been largely superseded by the straightforward, symptom-based approach embodied in the *DSM-III-R*). Among symptoms of schizophrenia, loose associations are among the most difficult to describe or quantify, so when present, it is advisable to record verbatim examples. Loose associations occur not only in schizophrenia but also in advanced dementia, severe mania, psychotic

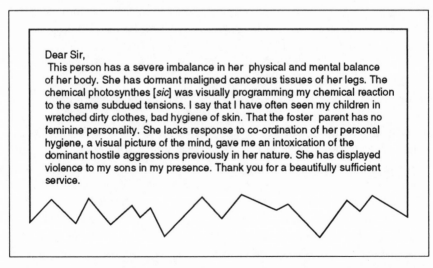

FIGURE 5–1   Excerpts from a letter by a schizophrenic patient demonstrating loose associations.

depression, drug intoxication or withdrawal, brief reactive psychosis, and delirium. Wernicke's aphasia should be distinguished from psychosis (see Chapter 4).

While loose associations are fairly common in psychotic and some brain-disordered patients, word salad and incoherence are much rarer. *Word salad* is an extreme form of loosening of associations named for its similarities to a tossed salad. Words are intact but are strung together with no apparent logical or meaningful connection. For example, "Print the light help for green ow mom don't wall and devil devil john green the african oh give green fun." The speech of a patient with word salad is fluent and prosodic compared to that in Broca's aphasia, but may be more difficult to distinguish from Wernicke's aphasia or severe Alzheimer's dementia. *Incoherence* is a less specific term than word salad and occurs in various disorders including delirium, dementia, aphasia, and severe manic psychosis. We prefer to use it to describe patients whose speech is truly unintelligible because of severe loosening of associations, poor articulation (dysarthria), or both. It is therefore preferable to elaborate other signs or symptoms in an incoherent patient in order to be more specific and aid in the differential diagnosis. An incoherent, actively psychotic schizophrenic patient is usually capable of comprehending commands, naming, repeating, reading, and writing, whereas delirious or fluently aphasic patients usually are not.

OTHER PECULIARITIES OF THOUGHT PROCESS
After assessing the organization of thinking, the examiner should indicate the presence of other peculiarities or specific derangements of thought process. These might include thought blocking, perseveration, clang associations, echolalia, or neologisms.

Thought blocking is a relatively rare phenomenon usually associated with psychosis and observed most frequently in schizophrenia and delirium. A thought is lost in midsentence, usually leading to a pause of a few seconds in speech. Blocking might be a phenomenon related to loose associations, in that when speech is resumed, the topic has changed. However, blocking is uniquely distinguished by the clear and unexpected pause between otherwise fluent statements. Blocking differs from the telegraphic speech of nonfluent aphasics in that in the former, pauses occur less frequently, conjunctives are not omitted, and grammar is intact. After blocking, the patient is generally unable to recollect the previous topic of conversation and is unaware that blocking occurred, as though thoughts had just "disappeared" from his or her mind. When normal individuals lose their train of thought, it can be distinguished from thought blocking by the overall context, awareness that the train of thought has been disrupted, recollection of the preceding topic, and the absence of loose associations. Histrionic patients may unconsciously block an affectively laden thought that is being repressed.

Perseveration is sometimes seen in psychosis, but is also seen in obsessive and brain-disordered patients (see Chapters 2 and 6). *Perseveration* refers to the nonvolitional repetition of verbal or motor activity. In the context of thought disorder, perseveration is the repetition of an idea, word, or phrase. Perseverative patients often seem mechanical or rote in their repetitiveness. In severe forms, such as in dementia, delirium, or catatonia, the same word or phrase is repeated frequently and out of context. In less severe cases, patients appear to have trouble "shifting gears" during the conversation; they appear stuck on a previous topic of conversation. For example, during an interview, a multiple sclerosis patient perseveratively repeated both his own and others' full names: "I am twenty-seven years old Dr. Robert Winfield Baker. I am from Pittsburgh, Dr. Robert Winfield Baker. Dr. Robert Winfield Baker is your name, is it not, Dr. Robert Winfield Baker?" This persisted throughout the entire interview.

In addition to those based on idiosyncratic meanings, examples of illogical associations include those based on sound. *Clang associations* are words or phrases that are connected by sound rather than by meaning; for example, "car–star–bar–guitar." Such associations are usually within the matrix of sentences: "I drive an old car. I wish upon a star. Do you drink in a bar? How do you play the guitar?" These illogical associations occur because of their similar sounds, unrelated to any meaningful connection.

Patients with *echolalia* repeat statements and questions made by the examiner, sometimes more than once. For example, when the examiner asks "What is today's date?" the patient replies "What is today's date?" Independently produced statements are scant or nonexistent. Fortunately this is a rare condition, seen most commonly in schizophrenia and mania, usually in association with catatonia (see Chapter 2). It also is seen in transcortical aphasias and in some patients with frontal dementias.

Novel, idiosyncratic words known as *neologisms* are evidence of psychosis (or possibly, of creativity). Examples are "I like the medicine, it gives me gisanesia" or "My frelox machine can cure schizophrenia" or "My mother stole my meurer." These occur in a minority of schizophrenic patients and are occasionally seen in other psychotic conditions, dementias, and aphasias. Neologisms are frequently rather elaborate yet plausible-sounding words; examiners should not hesitate to consult a dictionary and/or ask the patient to repeat, spell, or define a possible neologism. Psychotic patients who invent neologisms generally will not acknowledge that they have created them, but may happily spell them or define them ("Gisanesia is feeling good when you move your muscles"). Neologisms often are associated with delusions; for example, a grandiose patient may create terms to describe machines he has invented. Neologisms should be carefully differentiated from paraphasias (see Chapter 4).

PATIENT RECOGNITION OF ABNORMALITIES OF THOUGHT PROCESS
The identification of abnormalities of thought process permits the recognition of psychosis even in those patients who conceal their symptoms. In general, pa-

tients are not cognizant of thought process abnormalities and may react with anger or chagrin when the abnormalities are pointed out. An exception is a patient with flight of ideas who also acknowledges the associated racing thoughts. On the other hand, it is not uncommon for patients who have recovered from a psychotic episode or from delirium to describe how confused or mixed up they felt during the acute psychosis. More often, recovered delirious patients do not remember their thought-disordered period because they concurrently had impairment in their capacity to form new memories.

Schizophrenic patients sometimes think of their antipsychotic medication as something that "glues thoughts together." While such statements might first suggest delusional ideation, they really indicate a recognition of thought disorganization and a simplified description of the therapeutic action of medications. When able to gain awareness to the extent that the patient realizes his or her thinking was abnormal, and therefore undesirable, the symptom is termed *ego-dystonic*. In the absence of the patient's insight that a symptom is abnormal, it is termed *ego-syntonic* (see Insight, in Chapter 7).

Thought Content

The content of thought is a key diagnostic parameter that is assessed throughout the interview. The adept interviewer uses both careful listening and close questioning to assess the thought content. Special attention should be paid both to the opening minute of the examination and to any unstructured moments during the interview. These times offer particular opportunities to understand better what is on patients' minds: What do they see as the problems; why are they seeking help; and what do they bring up spontaneously? Some information about these questions is generally gained if the interview is initiated with open-ended questions. The unstructured portion of the interview allows one to gauge the organization of thought and to learn more about what themes are important to the patient. Overly structured or directive interviewers tend to miss these data and risk frustrating the patient. Sample opening questions include "What brings you here today?" "What kinds of problems have you been having?" "Tell me a little about yourself?" or "What have things been like since I last saw you?" In general, the patient should be given one to several minutes for spontaneous exposition (if so inclined), followed by requests for clarification or elaboration. If a patient proves too disorganized, too confused, or too anxious to handle open-ended questions or to speak spontaneously, a more directive approach becomes necessary. For example, a patient may be put at ease or allowed to "warm up" with a number of straightforward questions, such as "What is your name?" "Where do you live?" "Who do you live with?" or "How old are you?"

In most cases, the interviewer should explore in some depth the problems mentioned by the patient in the initial minutes of the examination. Elaboration, clarification, and quantification (how bad and for how long) provide informa-

Table 5.2. Important abnormalities
of thought content and perception

Thoughts	Percepts
Delusion	Autoscopy
Homicidal ideation	Déjà vu
Magical thinking	Depersonalization
Obsession	Derealization
Overvalued idea	Hallucination
Paranoia	Illusion
Phobia	Jamais vu
Poverty of speech	
Preoccupation	
Rumination	
Suicidal ideation	
Suspiciousness	

tion, communicate to the patient the examiner's interest in the problem, and afford an opportunity to observe thought content and process. It is advisable to consider the initial complaints closely, even if they seem delusional or unimportant.

Explicit inquiries should be made to delineate the general themes of the patient's thought content. Questions might include "What has been on your mind?" "Are there things that you've been worrying about?" "What is most important to you?" "What do you think about when you are alone/daydreaming/lying awake in bed?" If a patient seems distracted or unusually emotional, it is often profitable to inquire "What were you just thinking about?" to elicit the most active thought.

In an initial evaluation of a new patient, the examiner should ask a series of specific questions, analogous to the review of systems in the medical history. (During the review of systems, specific inquiries are made about each bodily system, e.g., respiratory, genitourinary, skin, and so on.) In this way, information that the patient did not realize was important can be uncovered. A psychiatric review of systems includes questions regarding the presence of several specific abnormalities of thought content, such as delusions, violent ideation, obsessions, phobias, and mistaken perception (see Table 5–2). These are detailed in the following sections.

PATIENT RECOGNITION OF ABNORMALITIES OF THOUGHT CONTENT
Not uncommonly patients come to psychiatric attention because of abnormal ideas, including delusions and obsessions. Abnormal ideas may distress the patient or those around the patient, often producing occupational or social disabili-

ty, and may even lead to aberrant or violent behavior. The level of the patient's insight, or awareness that thinking is abnormal, can significantly affect the elicitation of abnormal ideation during the examination. In terms of thought content, the degree of insight is related to the degree of recognition of reality. Reality includes both the external world and the individual's internal reality, as well as the capacity to be aware of both. Psychotic patients usually have impaired insight. By definition, delusions are not recognized by the patient as being false ideas or incongruent with reality. However, more insightful individuals may recognize the incongruity of their beliefs, using qualifiers like "I know it sounds strange but . . ." or "I had trouble believing it myself but . . ." Relatively insightful delusional patients often hide their delusions from the examiner in order to avoid some perceived consequence. For example, a patient remembers having been committed to the hospital every time he brings up his belief in a neighbor's murderous plot against him and, consequently, has learned to stop talking about the plot. Therefore, some degree of insight may render psychotic signs and symptoms more subtle, posing a greater challenge to the interviewer. On the other hand, partial insight is a sign of health: The patient can correctly interpret some aspects of reality. The patient's degree of awareness or insight can thus determine whether a symptom is ego-syntonic or ego-dystonic (see Chapter 7, Insight).

Abnormal thoughts may produce a variable emotional impact on the patient. Those who are distressed by the abnormal thoughts are much more likely to come to psychiatric attention. Patients who react to their delusions blandly (e.g., those with blunted affect, more common in chronic than in acute psychosis) or with pleasure (e.g., those with grandiose delusions of wealth, power, beauty, immortality, etc.) do not commonly seek treatment for their delusions. Contact, if initiated by the patient, occurs usually because of some other related symptom (trouble sleeping, mood disturbance); alternatively, it may occur because of a distressed third party (family), or even because of involuntary commitment. The need for involuntary hospitalization epitomizes a lack of insight into one's problems.

DELUSIONS

Delusions are objectively incorrect beliefs that are not culturally determined or shared with a large group of people (although shared delusions can occur) and that cannot be shaken by contrary evidence. Delusions can range from being quite bizarre and fragmented to being plausible and organized. In any case, labeling a statement as delusional requires judgment on the part of the examiner, a task more difficult when the delusions are mild and plausible. Such cases often provoke controversy, and students with little clinical experience at times take umbrage at labeling anything delusional unless it is extremely bizarre. In such situations, it is fair to take the whole clinical picture into account, including past history, when evaluating the accuracy of the patient's statements. For example, one may never be able to ascertain incontrovertibly that a patient is not a high-ranking CIA officer in hiding from foreign agents, though its likelihood of being delusional is high in a chronically institutionalized patient. In less clear cases, bets are hedged by referring to "possible delusions" in the written MSE. The adept examiner is simultaneously humble and confident—confident that mental illness does occur, that some individuals are delusional, and that delusions can be recognized for what they are. Yet the examiner should remain humble in the awareness that he or she is not the final arbiter of reality, and therefore needs to seek supporting evidence before calling something delusional (or when deciding that something is not delusional).

Apparent delusions should be evaluated in a societal and cultural context; unusual or bizarre ideas and beliefs may not be delusional if they are shared with a large group. Many religious tenets would strike a given examiner of a different religion as implausible (e.g., that humans are reincarnated as animals or that a piece of bread contains the body of Christ), yet are clearly not delusional. (Also, whereas some religious beliefs are literally held, other beliefs are recognized as symbolic.) Most religious beliefs are culturally determined, accepted, shared, and not the product of individual mental illness. On the other hand, delusions with a religious content are quite common, and religious cults and extreme sects are attractive to some mentally ill people. For example, a previously nonreligious person who suddenly becomes a religious zealot may have temporal lobe epilepsy, and manic or schizophrenic patients not uncommonly believe that they are divine. There are also nonreligious customs or beliefs that appear objectively impossible and unshakable, but nonetheless are not delusional. A common example in the southern United States is a belief in *rooting*, which involves a conviction that an evil spell can be cast. The examiner's task becomes more difficult as the size of the group that shares a possible delusion decreases, such as to a family unit or cult group. *Folie-à-deux* is a delusion shared by two individuals. Such shared delusions usually point to pathology of both the affected individuals and their relationship.

Psychotic patients can appear quite normal, and the presence of hallucinations or delusions can be readily missed by a superficial or presumptive examiner. Continual monitoring for delusions is necessary during treatment of psychotic patients as well as patients with disorders that may be associated with delusions, such as drug or alcohol abuse, dementias, delirium, and bipolar disorder. Initial diagnostic interviews should include careful attention to any clues to potential delusions, while seeking detailed clarification or elaboration of suggestive statements. For example, a statement that "my neighbors are always bothering me" should neither be accepted as factual (even if the examiner's neighbors are also bothersome) nor written down as a paranoid delusion. Instead, questioning should focus on in what way and to what degree the neighbors are bothersome, how certain the patient feels about it, on what evidence it is based, what the patient sees as the neighbors' motivation (to uncover persecutory feelings), and how the patient might revise his or her conclusion if contradictory evidence were to come to light. If available, family members or other involved parties may be able to clarify whether a particular statement is delusional. Corroborative history is often extremely valuable in the assessment of psychiatric patients, and particularly when evaluating the reality of questionably delusional statements.

Finally, a full evaluation should include specific questions to exclude the presence of the more common delusions, such as of being in danger, being watched, being plotted against, being discussed by the media, or having thoughts read.

The response of the examiner to reported delusions is a matter of individual style and will not be discussed in detail here. However, we do recommend that the examiner take a neutral approach during an initial interview, avoiding either supporting or contradicting apparent delusions. Information is gathered and active interest is conveyed by questioning to clarify and elicit the full extent of any delusions. On the other hand, helping patients to recognize the unreality of delusions is sometimes the goal of therapy and may alleviate distress or abort a violent plan. Even during a first evaluation, it may be helpful to challenge delusions in order to assess how fixed or unshakable they are, though this is usually more effective when done indirectly, for example, "Does your family feel the same way? Why not?" or "Could you be mistaken about this?" Not uncommonly, patients will ask the examiner's opinion about apparently delusional material. Delusional individuals are usually resistant to direct challenges of their beliefs, will deny the truth of evidence that contradicts the delusion, and may become angered or less communicative when confronted. Therefore, in initial interviews, we usually avoid answering queries as to our opinion about delusional matters, replying instead: "I need more information to comment" or "That's not something that I can be completely certain about."

Types. The first level of classification of delusions is by content. The most frequently encountered type is *paranoid*, which should be divided into the more specific categories of persecutory and grandiose delusions. *Schneiderian symptoms* include a number of delusions, such as thought control, that may be seen in severe psychotic disorders (see Definitions). Other important types of delusions are somatic, erotomanic, referential, nihilistic, and delusional denial.

Paranoid delusions include both grandiose and persecutory ones. *Persecutory* delusions are of harm or threats: "My medicine contains female hormones that are castrating me." "The psychiatrists have built machines that are projecting voices into my mind," "My boss is having me watched," "The other patients were planted here to spy on me," "My neighbors are trying to have me killed." Patients may also be guarded and vigilant or describe pervasive mistrust in the absence of any clear delusion. Such patients can be described as suspicious. Persecutory delusions are the most frequently encountered type of delusion in general psychiatric practice, including in delirious and demented patients. They may also be seen following right-hemispheric brain damage and in association with temporalimbic epilepsy.

Grandiose delusions, also known as delusions of grandeur, are false beliefs about extraordinary talents, prowess, or importance. Patients may claim to have millions of dollars in the bank, jewels in the museum, irresistible sexual attractiveness, ability to play any musical instrument well, friendships with the mayor, governor, president, or pope, or an expectation that they will save the world. In addition, patients may report that they are or are related to or involved with a famous person, often Jesus Christ, but also famous entertainers, politicians, or criminals. Although grandiose delusions are most common in mania, they can occur in other psychotic conditions and in chronic meningoencephalitis, particularly tertiary neurosyphilis. Delusions of poverty are the converse of some grandiose delusions; patients will insist that they are destitute and deny ownership of any of their assets.

Schneiderian symptoms are named for the psychiatrist who grouped them. *First-rank* Schneiderian symptoms were previously considered pathognomonic of schizophrenia, and remain important to contemporary diagnostic criteria, as embodied in *DSM-III-R*. These symptoms include a feeling that one is being externally controlled ("made" or "passivity" experiences), thought broadcasting, thought insertion or thought withdrawal, and certain hallucinatory experiences including commands or an ongoing commentary on one's behavior. *Thought broadcasting* is the belief that one's thoughts are no longer private; this is the most common Schneiderian symptom. Patients with thought broadcasting may repetitively apologize or say "I didn't mean that," as though the examiner could hear the [apparently derogatory] thought that the patient was experiencing. *Thought insertion* is the conviction that a thought is alien and placed in one's mind by some external power. *Thought withdrawal* is the delusional sense that thoughts are being lost or stolen through the efforts of some external force. Patients are frequently capable of elaborating their delusional conceptions of the source or cause of the Schneiderian symptom.

Erotomania is an ungrounded conviction that another person is deeply in love with oneself; for example, a woman believes that a relatively unapproachable man is covertly and deeply smitten by her. The erotomanic object is often a famous person, such as a television talk-show host. A previously asymptomatic college student, working as a corporate office assistant, suddenly perceived that an older executive was in love with her. This realization contained elements of delusions of reference (see below) in that she felt that correspondence assigned to her for typing contained an obscure code that confirmed the executive's love. She approached him several times, on one occasion, after breaking into his home. The patient's belief that this man loved her remained unswayed for several years despite her being fired, arrested, and committed to a hospital. She blamed these untoward events on the executive's wife. Erotomania is sometimes referred to as Clerambault's syndrome, as are other wholly unrelated phenomena. Eponyms can be confusing and are best avoided.

Delusional jealousy is virtually the inverse of erotomania; it is the unfounded and preoccupying conviction that one's spouse or lover is being unfaithful. Such patients may violently act on their delusions. Delusional jealousy is sometimes considered to be a type of persecutory delusion.

Reduplicative paramnesia or *delusional misidentification* can involve place, other persons, or self (including body parts). The fixed delusion that one is located elsewhere, such as at home rather than a hospital (reduplicative paramnesia for place), can occur in functional psychotic disorders, but is perhaps more common in amnestic states. The fixed belief that an imposter, often malevolent, has been substituted for one or more persons with whom the patient interacts (reduplicative paramnesia for person) is known as *Capgras' syndrome*. The substituted person is usually someone important to the patient, typically the spouse, and it is a selective delusion; that is, most people in the environment are correctly identified. Some have suggested that this phenomenon is related to *prosopagnosia* (inability to recognize faces), but patients with Capgras' syndrome are actually unimpaired in objective testing of facial recognition. Thus, it is a fixed delusion, a belief in the existence of the alleged double, as opposed to an illusion, hallucination, or misperception; it also is not due to diffuse cognitive deficits or amnesia. Whereas Capgras' syndrome involves the delusion that intimates have been replaced by strangers, schizophrenic patients often describe the converse, that strangers (such as other patients on the ward) are actually friends, relatives, or familiar persons from their past. To our knowledge, there is no eponym or other special name for this particular delusion; presumably it also occurs nonspecifically in various psychotic illnesses.

Reduplicative phenomena involving body parts (e.g., extra limbs or heads) are possibly delusions but more likely hallucinations or illusions, are typically transient (i.e., not "fixed"), and are likely to occur in confused patients and/or in response to acute neurologic injury, such as to the nondominant parietal lobe.

Somatic delusions are usually of being ill, but may be of some unusual bodily attribute. These delusions range from the plausible ("I have a broken arm") to the absurd or bizarre ("There are snakes in my heart"; "My brain is missing"). Narcissistically preoccupied patients may report that some feature of their appearance is particularly ugly (e.g., facial moles that are not objectively visible). Such delusions should be carefully evaluated, especially as they may contain a grain of reality or be based on a distorted report of a real pain or discomfort ("The medicine is rotting my intestines"). Mentally retarded persons may explain real somatic symptoms in fantastical ways. Somatic delusions must also be differentiated from conversion disorder or hypochondriasis; because plausible somatic delusions are sometimes termed *hypochondriacal delusions*, misdiagnosis could potentially result. Somatic delusions may accompany schizophrenia, brief reactive psychosis, major depression, dementia, delirium, or mania. Needless to say, before attributing a somatic complaint to a psychotic origin, a careful physical examination and appropriate laboratory testing need to be pursued.

The theme of *nihilistic delusions* is that some dire event is impending or, more likely, has taken place, such as that one is dead, has lost all possessions, has lost internal organs, is in need of burial, or is damned. The outside world does not exist or does not matter. Such delusions are also sometimes labeled delusions of negation or *Cotard's syndrome*. Capgras described a woman who felt her nothingness so emphatically that she called herself "Madame Zero."

Not uncommonly, psychotic patients assert that some personal attribute has been stolen or substituted; for example, they may claim a different name or a different family; that their sex or race has been changed; or that their brain, genitals, or heart have been stolen or substituted. Such delusions can have elements of persecutory, somatic, reduplicative, or nihilistic delusions.

A *referential delusion* is the incorrect ascription of special individual meaning to neutral stimuli. Such thoughts may be straightforward ("I am the hit-and-run driver that they've been discussing on TV") or quite idiosyncratic ("The red and black clothing on the mannequin in the local shop window is the signal that I am a sinner"). Referential thinking often relates to books, television, movies, radio, or newspapers; thus it is sometimes productive to ask the patient if he or she has noted anything about himself in any of these media: "Have you been getting any special messages from T.V. or radio?" Referential delusions are often termed *ideas of reference.*

Delusional denial is the rejection of some aspect of reality, even when confronted with clear evidence. The term *denial* is often used in general medical settings to describe patients' failure to accept what the doctor thinks is necessary, such as dieting, stopping smoking, or taking medication. In more extreme forms, denial may be of delusional proportions, such as people who temporarily reject the reality of a loss: "Don't take my mother away, she can't be dead!" Or "That's not my chart. I don't have cancer." This term can also be applied to the rejection by delusional patients of evidence that their delusions are not true. See Chapter 7 for further discussion of denial and associated defense mechanisms.

The term *bizarre* is also used to describe certain delusions and connotes that the delusion is totally implausible. For example, a patient believes he was born on Mars, chopped into pieces, transported to Earth a millennium ago, and then reassembled. On the other hand, because it is not inconceivable that the CIA, KGB, or Mafia might follow people, a delusion of being trailed by one of these organizations cannot be described as bizarre. The term bizarre can be used as an adjective for many of the descriptive terms already described; for example, a persecutory delusion may or may not be bizarre.

Monosymptomatic delusions are restricted to one delimited topic and occur in the absence of other gross psychopathology such as hallucinations. Their diagnostic, prognostic, and treatment implications may differ from those of other delusions. Classically they are of somatic symptoms, such as of something foreign under the skin. A patient may be convinced of having fleas, scratch himself, and use the excoriated areas as evidence of infestation. They can be of other types, however; for example, isolated erotomanic or jealous delusions are not uncommonly described as monosymptomatic.

Diagnostic Significance. The presence of delusions demonstrates the presence of a psychotic illness but does not necessarily distinguish the underlying disorder. Until well into this century, it was felt that certain types of delusions (Schneiderian symptoms) were pathognomonic of schizophrenia. Clinical observation with careful diagnostic formulation has demonstrated that each of these Schneiderian symptoms may occur in many other types of psychosis, such as in mania or delirium. Therefore, the diagnostic meaning of the type of delusion is only relative. Schneiderian symptoms are less commonly seen in affective psychoses; instead, one tends to expect persecutory, somatic, and nihilistic delusions in psychotic depression, and grandiose or persecutory delusions in mania. This expectation has resulted in the concept of mood-congruent or mood-incongruent delusions. *Mood congruency* means that the content of the delusion matches the patient's affective state—for example, the manic patient who believes that he is a multimillionaire and is irresistibly attractive to his psychiatrist and other women. *Mood-incongruent delusions* (e.g., thought broadcasting in a depressed patient) are a poor prognostic sign, and, in fact, may signal the need to reevaluate the diagnosis; that is, does the patient truly have an affective disorder, or is a schizophreniform disorder more likely? Mood congruency is a concept distinct from ego-syntonicity, which is discussed in this chapter above.

Although they are a hallmark of schizophrenia and other functional psychotic conditions, delusions may be manifestations of neurologic disease. For example, while reduplicative paramnesias are reported in schizophrenia and other psychotic disorders, they are seen commonly also in chronic or resolving amnestic syndromes (perhaps induced by closed head injury, dementia, or a confusional state). Sometimes reduplicative paramnesia occurs in the context of identifiable brain lesions; frontal, limbic, and right-hemispheric areas have all been implicated.

Organization and Consistency. Delusions vary in the degree that they are organized or systematized. Chronically psychotic patients usually have a stable set of delusions in which various psychotic features tend to interrelate, new symptoms are added to the matrix of old ones, and the patient is able to discuss most things in terms of his or her delusional system. Such delusions are appropriately labeled *stable* or *systematized*. For example, an elderly female patient with schizophrenia experiences continual derogatory auditory hallucinations of voices of her family members because they have a machine that broadcasts to a receiver that her previous physicians implanted in her brain. She feels that her family is maintaining her commitment to the hospital in order to prevent her access to the machine and that when she has a headache, it is due to the receiver in her brain. From time to time, she insists on a change of doctors when she "discovers" that her present doctor is involved in perpetuating the cruel functions of the machine. Another example is a hospitalized patient who believes that he is working undercover for the military. He feels that various staff members are either planted by the military to assist him or are members of opposing forces. He feels that his mission is to help the other patients and that related plans are being perfected in the military's lab for novel and bizarre machinery to cure the others. While initially resistant to a proposed discharge to a personal care home, he one day announces that he received military transfer orders, and would be stationed at the personal care home for 18 years. His delusions are systematized in that they are elaborate and consistent, and neatly envelop new circumstances or new acquaintances.

Unstable or *nonsystematized delusions* are those that change rapidly in content; their organization is difficult to elucidate, and the psychotic elements are not particularly interrelated. Although there is great overlap, stable and systematized delusions are seen most frequently in chronic, well-established conditions, whereas unstable, poorly systematized delusions tend to be more common in transient organic states (especially delirium) or at the time of onset of a psychotic condition. Of course, patients with thought process disorganization also are prone to have poor organization of any delusions.

Emotional and Behavioral Impact. Elucidating the content of delusions is also important in understanding the patient's feelings and behaviors. Many schizophrenic patients have a blunted affect, even showing little emotional response to their delusional beliefs. Nevertheless, delusions may be quite terrifying to the psychotic patient. In this context, it is not surprising that individuals can act on the basis of their delusions, and sometimes quite violently (fortunately, rarely). There have been homicides by paranoid persons who kill to forestall a perceived danger; accidental deaths of those who behave recklessly because of delusions of immortality; suicides in response to guilty or nihilistic delusions; and self-mutilation because of somatic delusions. Though violent behavior cannot always be predicted, elucidation of the content of delusions may herald possible risk.

NEAR-DELUSIONAL BELIEFS

Overvalued ideas are thoughts that cannot be called delusional with certainty. These are ideas that are odd, not mainstream, and firmly held, but not sufficiently absurd, illogical, or unshakable to warrant a delusional label. Alternatively, qualifiers such as likely, possible, or questionable can be used when there is uncertainty whether or not a particular idea is delusional.

Magical thinking is illogical, often attributing more connectedness to events than is actually the case; many superstitions are examples of culturally validated magical thinking. Individual examples might include the belief that donating money to charities will make the boss grant a raise or that an extramarital affair was responsible for a traffic accident. Such thinking is common among children and obsessive-compulsive or schizophrenic patients, and is not necessarily indicative of psychopathology.

OBSESSIONS AND PREOCCUPATIONS

Obsessions are undesired, unpleasant, intrusive thoughts that cannot be suppressed through the patient's own volition. They are typically, but not necessarily, persistent and frequent. They are frequently concurrent with compulsions, which are discussed in Chapter 2. Although the patient realizes that the obsessions are unreasonable, they cannot be suppressed or ignored. Sometimes the obsession is a single word or phrase that keeps recurring; more frequently it is a recurrent theme. Common themes are of engaging in some violent, silly, or socially inappropriate behavior. For example, a patient may keep feeling that he will poison the city's water supply; or that he will rape and murder women like a modern Jack the Ripper; or that he will shout obscenities during church services. Patients view such behaviors as abhorrent and are distressed by their thoughts, but cannot stop thinking them. These are not true homicidal thoughts, and obsessive patients are generally not dangerous to others, as they recognize the thoughts as absurd and have no intent or plan to act on them; actually, they desperately want not to do these things (see inhibiting obsessions, below). Such obsessions are not delusions and are distinguishable from delusions by the presence of insight (see Chapter 7).

Obsessions are sometimes categorized into subtypes. A *ruminative obsession* (also called *intellectual obsession*) involves metaphysical or philosophical thoughts, such as the purpose of life or the fate of mankind. The appellation is derived from the cow's technique of regurgitating and rechewing its food, called rumination. These thoughts are mulled over continually without resolution.

With a *doubting obsession*, patients cannot stop thinking about some decision that has to be made or that has been made. Unfortunately, all alternatives (and especially the negative aspects of each potential choice) are weighed ad nauseam without reaching a conclusion. While these doubting obsessions may involve important decisions, they are more often about something trivial—for example, what to eat, what to wear, what route to take. (In fact, it is quite normal to worry moderately over, or second-guess, major decisions like getting married or divorced, buying a house, changing jobs, etc.) In a severe form, doubting obsessions are incapacitating.

Inhibiting obsessions often involve violent ideation, as in raping or poisoning others. Such patients do not experience a real urge to commit such crimes, but instead repeatedly experience fear or premonition of committing these acts. The patient usually recognizes that the obsessive thoughts are unrealistic. Nevertheless, the patient may become incapacitated (inhibited) and isolated as he or she does nothing at all for fear of losing control and acting violently.

A key feature of obsessive thoughts is that they are unwanted and as such are ego-dystonic or ego-alien. Many people can have unpleasant or extremely repetitive thoughts, but they are not truly obsessions unless they are unwanted and unsuppressible. For example, patients will be encountered who think most of the time about one theme (money, death, sex, a hobby, etc.), but if they want to think about this or can exclude the theme from conscious thought, they have preoccupations rather than obsessions. *Preoccupations* are undue visitations to a topic, usually communicated by a persistent return to that topic during conversation. Common preoccupations include health concerns, physical appearance, finances, romance, and sex. However, patients can also be preoccupied with their psychiatric symptoms, such as their delusions or hallucinations.

Examination for Obsessions. Like most signs and symptoms, the examiner uncovers obsessions through observation and questioning. "Are there any repetitive thoughts that bother you or that you can't stop?" "Do you have any impulses that you want to stop but can't?" Patients who seem preoccupied with one theme should be closely questioned regarding possible obsessions. Obsessions and compulsions are more likely in patients whose overall thinking is rigid, stereotyped, and repetitive; in those who are fastidious, perfectionistic, and very concerned about time; and in those who rearrange the environment (even if it is *your* office). If possible obsessions or preoccupations are uncovered, questioning should focus on their content and frequency. It is very important to ascertain whether they are unwanted, whether the patient has tried to stop them, how they affect the patient's life, and whether they cause any actions or compulsions.

Diagnostic Significance. Obsessions and preoccupations can be seen in a variety of clinical states. Normal individuals have varying degrees of thoughts and behaviors that appear obsessive or compulsive, and these tend to be exaggerated under stress. Such behaviors can be adaptive and may be quite socially acceptable, such as great concern with punctuality, or a desire always to arrange the contents of drawers or shelves in a particular way. Such thoughts or actions cannot be labeled as obsessions or compulsions if the patient does not acknowledge that they are unwanted or ego-dystonic. Nevertheless, clinicians might record these as obsessive (or compulsive) traits or characteristics. These may be helpful descriptors of personality or personal style. Obsessive-compulsive behaviors and thoughts that are not unwanted by the patient and not maladaptive are not necessarily indicative of psychopathology. An alternative approach is to describe them in the Appearance, Attitude, and Activity section of the MSE: "The patient is very neatly dressed and repeatedly adjusted his clothing and coiffure during the interview"; or "The patient repeatedly checked his watch and asked many times about the length of the appointment, the time and duration of the next appointment, etc." Normal individuals may also display preoccupations with major decisions or problems that they are facing. This can be noted for the sake of description, but is not indicative of the presence of mental illness.

Obsessions (and compulsions) may be associated with obsessive-compulsive disorder, anxiety, mood disorder, psychoses, and organic mental disorders. Because obsessions are usually considered anxiety symptoms, elicitation of other signs or symptoms of anxiety should be undertaken. Obsessions may also be a prodromal sign of impending psychosis: Schizophrenics sometimes exhibit strange and ritualistic behaviors. Patients with depression commonly have obsessive, though rarely compulsive, features, especially ruminative obsessions. Moreover, those with obsessive-compulsive disorder seem predisposed to depression; therefore, the presence of obsessive symptoms is also an indication to seek the presence of an affective disorder. Although these symptoms occur more rarely as manifestations of a neurologic disorder, they are seen in Tourette's disease, Huntington's disease, postencephalitic parkinsonism, basal ganglia damage from anoxia or carbon monoxide poisoning, and in strokes, tumors, or seizures affecting basal ganglia or limbic areas.

PHOBIAS

A *phobia* is a dread of an object or situation that does not in reality pose any threat. Phobic patients are not delusional; they intellectually recognize that there is no danger. This intellectual recognition unfortunately does not prevent their emotional response of fear. Phobias are divided into three groups: agoraphobia, social phobia, and simple phobias.

The term *agoraphobia* is derived from a Greek term which refers to the open marketplace. Most agoraphobic patients fear not only open spaces but also all public places, or particular public places (e.g., a certain store or street, any place that is crowded, elevators, etc.), regardless of whether these places are open. As a consequence, these patients may become homebound. Panic attacks (see Chapter 3) are a frequent and severe complication of agoraphobia. Symptoms of *panic* include a sense of impending doom, and evidence of autonomic hyperactivity, such as sweating, palpitations, or hyperventilation. In addition, agoraphobia is complicated by social and simple phobias (see immediately below), dysphoria, anxiety, obsessions (see this chapter, above), and depersonalization (see this chapter, below). Agoraphobia is probably the most common of the phobias and is the most debilitating.

A *social phobia* is the fear of public humiliation. Social phobia most often focuses on public speaking. A variety of other potentially embarrassing circumstances may underlie a social phobia, such as fear of blushing, fear of fainting, or fear of financial discussions. Some judgment is required by the examiner in drawing a line between normal social sensitivity and social phobia. In fact, concern over how one's appearance or actions are perceived by others is normal to the extent that an absence of social attentiveness is considered rude and possibly pathologic (e.g., narcissistic or schizoid personality disorders). In the MSE, findings suggestive of social phobia should be recorded if the patient is complaining of them, if they significantly interfere with the patient's social or occupational functioning, if the fears are much more powerful than in most people, or if the fears are provoked by social situations that should not be at all stressful for most people.

The classification *simple phobias* covers all other phobic symptoms. A simple phobia is a circumscribed but inordinate fear of a particular situation or object. Fear of blood, heights, flying, closed spaces, spiders, dogs, or bodies of water are all common phobias; the possible types of simple phobias are almost limitless. Those phobias that focus on a social interaction—for example, speaking to a person of the opposite sex—should be classified as social phobias. Simple phobias are not usually indicators of severe psychopathology, but may have a specific behavioral impact, such as needing to travel by trains rather than airplanes. Children are especially prone to phobias. A phobic patient may have more than one phobic stimulus, that is, fear more than one type of object or situation. Patients should be closely questioned about their phobias in order to ensure that they recognize that their fears are idiosyncratic rather than provoked by a realistic danger; this reality testing differentiates phobias from persecutory delusions or magical thinking.

Phobic patients, especially those who have panic attacks, can become quite anxious simply by thinking about encountering their phobic stimulus. Such *anticipatory anxiety* may be observed during the interview.

VIOLENT IDEATION (SUICIDAL AND HOMICIDAL)
Ideation of violence toward self or others is one of the most important areas of thought content for assessment in the MSE. The MSE report should document the presence or absence of suicidal and violent ideation and some assessment of its severity or urgency.

Suicidal ideation varies in its intensity. Even more common than active suicidal intent is ideation about one's own death and its consequences. Some patients have *passive death wishes*—that is, a desire to die without any specific intent actively to harm themselves. Some consider killing themselves but have no specific plan. In many patients, the desire or ideation about suicide is really a desire to escape their situation or problems. For others, suicide represents a desperate attempt to exercise some control in their troubled lives or is an expression of their anger toward others whom they want to make feel guilty, manipulate, or gain revenge against.

Actively suicidal patients are those who intend to die and are contemplating specific plans for committing suicide. Such plans may involve shooting, hanging, carbon monoxide poisoning, drug overdoses, intentional car accidents, or jumping from a high place. Suicidal patients in general hospitals are more likely to jump from a window, whereas those in psychiatric hospitals are more likely to hang themselves. Even in a protected environment with suicide precautions in effect, such as a locked psychiatric ward, a patient intent on killing him- or herself may find a way.

While patients with chronic schizophrenia or recurrent mood disorders have a greater risk of dying by suicide than the general population, anxiety disorders, organic states, and drug and alcohol abuse also have an associated risk of suicide. Alcoholics more commonly attempt suicide while intoxicated. Even delirious patients can kill themselves, usually accidentally. Manic patients sometimes kill themselves as a result of recklessness, abrupt swings into depression, or psychosis. Schizophrenic patients kill themselves for a variety of reasons, including response to overwhelmingly terrify[ing] [de]lusions, delusions of invulnerability, command hallucinations, or concur[rent] [mood] [depression]. On the other hand, homicide by psychiatric patients is less co[mmon] [than] in the general population and much less common than suic[ide] [in] [psychiatric] [p]atients, but nevertheless should be assessed, particularly in a [history or p] [p]atients.

Although suicide is a rar[e] [event] [that] [is] [stati]stically speaking, not possible to predict, there are some ris[k] [factors] which have retrospectively been associated with successful [suicides] [inc]lude a past history of suicide at-tempts, depression, sever[e] [substance] abuse, male gender, white race, advanced age, and a ch[ronic] [or] [serious] [phy]sical illness. Women attempt suicide about three times [often] [as] [men] [m]en actually kill themselves about twice as often as women because [they] [ten]d to use less lethal means, such as drug overdoses, whereas men more often choose guns. Knowing those features associated with completed suicides may guide the assessment of suicidality.

Inexperienced physicians erroneously may avoid discussing suicidality because of a concern that they may "put the thought" into the mind of a patient who had not previously considered it. To the contrary, psychiatric patients are often grateful for the opportunity to discuss their suicidal thoughts. Suggested questions for exploring suicidal ideation include the following: "Are there times when it seems like these problems are too much for you to bear?" "Do you ever find yourself thinking that you would be better off dead?" "Does life seem to be devoid of pleasure?" "Does it feel as if life is no longer worth living?" "Have you wished that you could die?" "Do you have thoughts about taking your own life?" If the patient acknowledges death wishes or suicidal thoughts, the physician should determine when these thoughts occurred, whether they included suicidal intent or any specific plan, the details of the plan, and whether the patient has taken any steps to further the plan, such as purchasing a lethal weapon or arranging financial affairs (writing a will, adjusting beneficiaries of life insurance policies, leaving a note, etc.). If the patient has not yet acted upon the thoughts, questioning should focus on how he or she handled them, whether he or she sought support from loved ones, called a hotline, and so on. Elaboration of these details should also be documented in the history of present illness because it serves as a basis for clinical interventions to protect the patient's safety (including, if necessary, involuntary hospitalization), and as a medicolegal document in the event of a clinical care review or a lawsuit.

Self-mutilation without intent to die is seen most frequently in patients who have primitive personality disorders and schizophrenia. Self-abusive acts, typically superficial cuts and burns, are a hallmark of the borderline personality disorder. These chronically self-abusive and/or suicidal patients make repeated self-destructive *gestures* related to manipulating interpersonal relationships (or to counter feelings of derealization), as opposed to acting from a real intent to die. The risk factors for suicide that were discussed above do not apply to the *chronic suicidality* of personality-disordered patients. In contrast, self-mutilation in psychotic patients is generally not for manipulative purposes and is often more severe in nature—for example, autocastration in response to a delusion of being harmed by testosterone. Head shaving that occurs in psychotic patients is a possible prologue to further self-injury.

The bulk of serious violence in the United States is not perpetrated by psychiatric patients. *Ideation of violence* toward others should nonetheless be mentioned in the MSE. Individuals with antisocial personality disorder are notoriously deficient in their empathy for others and in their acceptance of societal or moral restrictions, so they may act in violent or cruel ways. Conduct-disordered children torture animals, set fires, beat up smaller children, and so on. Paranoid individuals sometimes act on their delusions with violent preemptory strikes; hence paranoid patients should be asked how they plan to deal with their fears and whether they have had thoughts of harming others. Those with brain injury affecting the prefrontal cortex are disinhibited and impulsive. Violence may occur in severely depressed and despondent individuals who sometimes commit so-called "murder suicides."

The physician should inquire whether the patient has ever harmed anyone, ever seriously injured another person such that medical treatment was necessary, or feels like hurting anyone currently or in the foreseeable future. Even though the clinician cannot predict homicide or assaultive behavior, it is important to document the presence or absence of *aggressive urges* or plans in the MSE. Commitment proceedings or police action may need to be initiated to deal with *actively homicidal* patients. Laws and precedents vary in each state regarding the duty to warn specific potential victims of homicidal ideas. A balance between the duties of patient confidentiality and protection of others is the crux of this issue; clinicians should educate themselves about laws and trends in their state.

Perception

Perceptual disturbances can take the form of hallucinations, illusions, derealization, depersonalization, autoscopy, déjà vu, or jamais vu. *Hallucinations* are unprovoked perceptual experiences that occur in the mind of the patient. They occur in any sensory modality (sight, hearing, smell, taste, touch) in the absence of any external physical stimulation, and may be simple or complex. Patients with chronic psychotic conditions may hallucinate continually. Other patients may have episodic or single-episode hallucinations, such as those induced by psychoactive drugs or those that accompany delirium.

In contrast to hallucinations, *illusions* are the exaggeration, distortion, or misinterpretation of an actual physical stimulus. Mirages of desert oases are visual illusions; hearing one's name in the noise of the wind blowing through trees is an auditory illusion. *Metamorphosia* is a visual illusion in which images of actual objects or persons are distorted in size (micropsia or macropsia) or shape, as experienced by Alice in Wonderland. *Micropsia* is the illusory perception of everything in the environment being unduly small, whereas in *macropsia* objects seem quite large. Visual perseveration or *palinopsia* is the persistence or repeated recurrence of something that was previously seen but is no longer within the field of vision. Patients with cortical blindness due to bilateral occipital lesions confabulate descriptions of what they cannot see (*Anton's syndrome*). Although illusions are not infrequent in psychosis, delirium, dementia, and neurologic disorders such as temporal lobe epilepsy, they also may occur in normal individuals.

Depersonalization is a feeling that one's self or one's body is unreal or unfamiliar. This includes a sense of being outside of one's self, that one's goals or mores are wrongheaded or meaningless; it is generally accompanied by anxiety or dysphoria. *Derealization*, the feeling that the world is unreal or has abruptly taken on unreal characteristics, is to the external environment what depersonalization is to the internal one. Patients describe feeling as though they are in a play or in outer space. Except in the most extreme cases, patients with depersonalization or derealization have the feelings of unreality, yet intellectually recognize what is or is not real. Thus, depersonalization and derealization are usually not delusional. Depersonalization and derealization are most commonly encountered in borderline personality disorder, partial complex seizure disorders, conversion or hysterical disorders, early or mild psychotic states, and normal adolescence. These experiences are usually transient, lasting minutes to hours, but may recur. Some patients experience both derealization and depersonalization.

Déjà vu is the perception of having previously seen or lived the current (novel) setting or situation. *Jamais vu* is more or less the converse: the sense that something familiar is strange, as though it is being seen or experienced for the first time. Both symptoms have been associated with complex partial epilepsy, but can occur in a variety of psychiatric and neurologic disorders, and, if of moderate or less degree, can be experienced by otherwise healthy persons.

Hallucinations occur in every sensory modality. Auditory hallucinations are characteristic of schizophrenia and mood disorders. Other forms of hallucina-

tions frequently coexist with auditory hallucinations in primary psychiatric disorders; however, the presence of other forms of hallucinations in the absence of the
auditory type is strongly suggestive of organicity. *Hypnagogic* hallucinations are
those that occur between wakefulness and falling asleep, whereas *hypnopompic*
hallucinations occur during the transition between sleep and awakening; they are
most commonly visual, occasionally auditory, and may be complex. Hypnagogic
and hypnopompic hallucinations appear to be dreamlike states and are not
necessarily indicative of psychopathology; rather, they are commonly associated
with narcolepsy.

Hallucinations are often closely related to delusions; for example, in alcoholic
hallucinosis, persecutory delusions that "explain" the voices often occur, such as
"the transmitter that was implanted in my head." In other cases it may be
difficult to determine if a particular report is delusional or hallucinatory, such as
a patient who complains that staff members are talking about him or her, or
another who says that her double is following her around. In such cases, the
examiner should clarify whether the patient actually sees or hears these things, or
instead knows of them through some other means.

AUDITORY HALLUCINATIONS

Auditory hallucinations are the most frequently encountered type of hallucination, and are particularly important in "primary" psychiatric illnesses. They can
range from elemental sounds to well-formed and elaborate conversations. In our
experience, clearly articulated voices are most frequently reported by psychotic
schizophrenic patients. If the voices give directives or instructions, they are
termed *command auditory hallucinations*. Auditory hallucinations are often
derogatory, insulting, or critical of the patient. Less commonly, the hallucination may be of more than one voice carrying on a conversation. Patients also
hear vague voices, indistinct sounds, or a buzzing or ringing in the ears. These
less distinct hallucinations are less valuable to establishing a diagnosis of schizophrenia. Hallucinations of buzzing or elemental sounds are more suggestive of a
neurologic problem (e.g., ear, acoustic nerve, or central auditory system pathology). In fact, ringing in the ears, or tinnitus, occurs with salicylate (aspirin)
intoxication. Formed *musical hallucinations* can occur in psychotic illnesses but
are also an infrequent concomitant of acquired deafness, particularly in those
with musical training and in patients with right temporal lobe epileptiform
discharges.

Some patients perceive hallucinated voices as originating within their heads,
whereas others perceive them as coming from outside, like normal conversation.
Although some consider the former to be relatively more healthy and/or insightful, this has not been established.

Certain types of auditory hallucinations are classified among the Schneiderian
symptoms (see above). These include auditory hallucinations of one or more

voices in a running commentary that remark on the patient's thoughts and behavior, or those of more than one voice conversing with one another.

VISUAL HALLUCINATIONS

Visual hallucinations occur in many mental disorders, often in conjunction with auditory hallucinations. Chronic visual hallucinations occur in Alzheimer's dementia and can be complex; for example, patients have described seeing people (who are not actually present) visiting and sitting on the living room sofa each day, or people coming into the kitchen and stealing all the food from the refrigerator. In addition to these complex, well-formed hallucinations, chronic visual hallucinations may also be poorly formed and described as flashing lights or colors; rarely are these distinct and frightening. *Autoscopic hallucinations* are the experience of seeing oneself, as though in a mirror, often secondary to temporal lobe seizures. *Lilliputian hallucinations* are of very tiny objects.

Visual hallucinations usually suggest "organicity"; that is, they occur as a result of dementia, delirium, recently developed blindness, drug withdrawal states (classically in delirium tremens, patients report seeing insects or animals), drug intoxications (especially with hallucinogenic, anticholinergic, or dopaminergic substances), temporal lobe epilepsy, migraine, and other organic mental disorders. Lesions of the thalamus and/or cerebral peduncles (i.e., areas not immediately involved in the geniculocalcarine or visual tract) can cause *peduncular hallucinations*, which are vivid, colorful, well-formed, but changeable images. Visual hallucinations may be accompanied by other evidence of delirium (such as fluctuating cognitive performance and level of consciousness) or of physical illness. Moderately abnormal visual experiences occur in ocular and neurologic diseases. For example, flashing lights occur with retinal detachment, whereas scintillating lights, a series of undulating jagged lines, blurred areas, or dark spots occur in migraine (*scotomas*). Seeing a curtain of darkness lower over the visual field is a sign of transient ischemic attack. Small dark specks, called floaters, that drift across the visual field are a common and benign result of senescent changes in the eye.

OTHER TYPES OF HALLUCINATIONS

Olfactory hallucinations are relatively rare and, like visual hallucinations, are quite suggestive of a neurologic problem. Olfactory hallucinations are rarely pleasant and are typically of a foul, stinking smell, such as burning rubber, feces, or rotting garbage. Epileptiform discharges in the temporal lobe are a common cause of olfactory hallucinations; they occur in isolation or as an aura preceding a secondarily generalized convulsion.

Gustatory (taste) *hallucinations* are the least frequently encountered type. Gustatory hallucinations are also usually associated with temporal lobe epilepsy and tend to be unpleasant.

Somatic hallucinations are of bodily sensations, most commonly on the surface of the skin, at which time they can be termed *tactile* or *haptic* hallucinations. *Formication* is the experience of ants crawling over one's skin, and is
particularly common in delirium tremens, delirium secondary to anticholinergic or other drug toxicity, and in delusions of parasitosis. Rarely, somatic
hallucinations are of an internal bodily sensation (*autonomic* or *cenesthetic* or
visceral hallucinations), which are difficult to distinguish from a somatic delusion (particularly if there is elaboration about their cause, such as "holes in my
heart" or "snakes in my bowels"). A common autonomic aura is the so-called
epigastric aura, a rising feeling originating in the abdomen and climbing to the
chest, throat, and/or mouth; this reflects a partial seizure involving the mesial
temporal region. Somatic hallucinations occur in psychosis and in neurologic
dysfunction. Moreover, a possible primary physical etiology in the involved
organ or body area should be investigated and excluded prior to ascribing an
abnormal perception to an hallucinatory experience. Bizarre somatic descriptions by schizophrenic patients may contain the clues to the authentic underlying pathology that could be missed by all except the most conscientious and
attentive physicians.

Evaluation for Hallucinations. Because patients do not always spontaneously
report hallucinations, the symptom may need to be inferred through close observation. Patients experiencing auditory hallucinations may pause during conversations and appear preoccupied while they are actually attending to hallucinations. Less frequently, they look toward the direction they perceive as the source
of the voice or vision, or even respond to the hallucination verbally or physically.
These behaviors are indirect clues, and, if appropriate to the situation, the
examiner may ask, "What was happening just then?" or "You seemed distracted
just now. Were you hearing someone else?"

A history of auditory hallucinations or evidence of active psychosis increases
the likelihood of current hallucinations. Virtually all patients should be asked at
some point during an initial evaluation whether they have experienced hallucinations. Hallucinations are common, even in superficially nonpsychotic individuals. Patients who are newly experiencing hallucinations are on average more
distressed by them as compared to those who have hallucinated chronically;
therefore, the latter group is less prone spontaneously to report them. Occasionally, hallucinations are covered up by patients who are paranoid or who recognize that acknowledgment of hallucinations can lead to hospitalization, increased medication, or some other undesired consequence. In such cases an
indirect approach is indicated. The issue may be defused by inquiring about past
rather than current symptoms, or by placing it in a broader context, such as, "It is
very common for people in your situation sometimes to hear voices even when
they can't see the person talking to them. Has this ever happened to you?" A

minority of patients will persist in denying the occurrence of hallucinations even while giving behavioral evidence of their presence (e.g., talking to an unseen person). The physician should document the patient's denial and the examiner's reasons suspecting their presence.

When hallucinations are acknowledged by any patient, the examiner should attempt to clarify their content. In the case of auditory hallucinations, it should be established whether more than one voice is heard, whether the voice is of someone known to the patient, and whether it is derogatory or critical. It is extremely important to ascertain whether command hallucinations are present, especially those urging violent or dangerous behavior. If command hallucinations are present, it should be determined whether the patient has acted on them and how difficult they are to resist.

To screen for nonauditory types of hallucinations, broad questions usually suffice, such as "Have you had other unusual sensory experiences like seeing things that aren't there, smelling things that aren't there, tasting something when there's nothing in your mouth, or feeling things that aren't real?" More detailed questioning is required if such symptoms are highly suspected, such as in patients with temporal lobe epilepsy.

Significance of Perceptual Disturbance. The presence of hallucinations helps establish the diagnosis of a psychotic illness. They may signal a primary psychotic illness such as schizophrenia, schizoaffective disorder, or brief reactive psychosis, or an illness with secondary or associated psychotic symptoms, such as depression, mania, delirium, Alzheimer's disease, amphetamine intoxication, and alcohol withdrawal.

Hallucinations in any modality other than auditory are suggestive of a neurologic or medical problem. If such hallucinations are present without auditory hallucinations, medical and neurologic evaluations should be done, even if the patient has been previously diagnosed with schizophrenia. (This is not to say that even auditory hallucinations should not be medically evaluated at some point.) Visual hallucinations occur in drug intoxication and withdrawal states, seizures, delirium, brain tumors, and so forth. Olfactory hallucinations are particularly suggestive of pathology in the temporal lobe/limbic area.

Definitions

Autoscopy The hallucinatory experience of seeing one's self.

Blocking The patient's speech and thought are interrupted in midsentence and do not resume their course. If patients are articulate about what is happening to them, they will often describe that "the idea disappeared from my head." This should be distinguished from a failure to answer owing to preoccupation with hallucinations.

Capgras' syndrome   The delusional conviction that a personally important individual (e.g., husband or wife) has been replaced by a stranger, an imposter. It is related to reduplicative paramnesia.

Circumstantiality   Talking at length around a point before finally getting to it, usually in an overly detailed fashion. The examiner may need to prod the patient to get to the point.

Clang associations   A form of loose associations in which statements are connected by sound and not by meaning (e.g., "station–nation–ablation"). The significance of this must be judged in broad context, because clang associations can occur in poetry, in addition to mental illnesses like mania and other forms of psychosis.

Delusional misidentification   See reduplicative paramnesia.

Déjà vu   The feeling that one has experienced a particular moment before. This impression of familiarity in an unfamiliar situation usually lasts a few seconds. Though present in many conditions like psychosis or borderline personality disorder and in normals, it is classically associated with partial complex seizure disorders.

Delusions   Objectively incorrect beliefs that are not culturally determined or shared with a large group and that cannot be shaken by contrary evidence. Systematized delusions are well organized and complex, have multiple elements around a central theme, and are relatively stable over time. Certain religious tenets may seem objectively incorrect and unshakable, but should not be considered delusional because they are culturally determined. Delusions are frequently the cornerstone of a diagnosis of psychosis, but certainly can be caused by neurologic as well as psychiatric disorders. There are many subcategories or specifically named delusions, some of which are defined as follows:

> *Grandiose*   A deluded belief that one possesses special wealth, powers, skill, influence, or destiny. Thought content that is indicative of unduly inflated self-esteem or exaggerated self-confidence may also be called "grandiose" without indicating that it is delusional. Grandiose delusions are thought to be "mood-congruent" and common in mania, but certainly occur in other psychotic conditions as well.

> *Nihilistic*   Belief that one is dead or empty or that some calamity is impending or has taken place; for example, the belief that the world is ending, or that God despises oneself.

> *Paranoid*   Used most commonly as a synonym for persecutory delusion. However, the word "paranoia" is important as a diagnostic term (e.g., in

paranoid disorder and paranoid schizophrenia), which can encompass symptoms other than persecutory feelings. Paranoid patients often have persecutory delusions, but may also have grandiose delusions or delusions of reference.

Persecutory The belief that one is being harmed, watched, ridiculed, manipulated, discriminated against, or plotted against, by another individual or group.

Somatic A delusion about some bodily abnormality, illness, or special attribute. These delusions may be straightforward convictions of illness, such as cancer or heart failure, but at times are bizarre, such as of snakes eating at organs or electrical wiring in the limbs. They are commonly associated with major depression, mania, and delirium, though more bizarre delusions tend to occur in schizophrenia.

Denial An inability or extreme reluctance to accept some aspect of reality even when it is demonstrated by another. Denial may be encountered in general medical practice: "My chest pain is just indigestion" or "Cigarettes won't hurt me." More severe forms may be seen in the face of a major trauma or in psychotic illnesses. Denial is to be differentiated from the psychologic defense mechanisms of repression, suppression, and rationalization. In these defenses, certain aspects of reality are avoided and excluded from conscious awareness, but on direct confrontation reality is not denied (see Chapter 7). Denial of a body part or dysfunction of a body part might indicate *anosognosia*. This is a form of psychotic denial, but typically occurs as a consequence of a well-defined neurologic lesion (see Chapter 7).

Depersonalization A feeling of unfamiliarity with oneself that is usually not delusional. Patients feel as though they are "outside" of themselves. Depersonalization should be differentiated from autoscopy (see *visual hallucination* in this section under Hallucination), in which patients actually see themselves, as if from some external vantage point in the room.

Derailment Thoughts are disconnected or illogically connected. Speech is difficult to follow because it jumps from one topic to another in a matter analogous to a train derailing or jumping off the tracks. This term also implies severe loosening of associations.

Derealization A feeling that the surrounding world has abruptly become unreal or taken on unreal qualities. As patients generally retain the recognition that this feeling is not true, derealization is seldom delusional.

Echolalia An uncommon disorder in which the subject repeats the statements of the examiner rather than speaking his or her own thoughts (see Chapter 4). It occurs in catatonia as well as in certain neurologic disorders.

Erotomania   A delusional belief that one is loved, perhaps secretly, by some other person.

Flight of ideas   A disorder in the connectedness of thought processes in which the patient's topic of conversation changes repeatedly, tangentially, and quickly, even from one sentence to the next. This is classically seen in mania, and therefore, many clinicians consider rapid, pressured speech (see Chapter 4) to be an integral part of flight of ideas. Flight of ideas is on a continuum with loosening of associations (see below in this section) at one extreme, and normal flow and connectedness at the other. In flight of ideas the logical connection between ideas is retained, whereas in loosening of associations the logical connection is lost.

Formal thought disorder   A disturbance of the structure or form of thought, as opposed to a disorder of thought content. This is not a particularly helpful term, and when used is usually synonymous with loosening of associations. However, tangentiality, perseveration, neologisms, and derailment are also examples of formal thought disorder.

Guardedness   Wariness and resistance to discussing personal matters, often accompanying suspiciousness and physical evidence of arousal and vigilance. Often seen in paranoid or delusional patients, but the term does not necessarily imply psychosis.

Hallucination   A perceptual disturbance that occurs as an internal thought in the absence of an external sensory stimulation. Each modality of sensation has a corresponding type of hallucination: auditory, visual, olfactory, gustatory, and tactile; and they may occur in combination. Functional psychosis is often accompanied by auditory hallucinations, sometimes along with hallucinations in other sensory spheres. The presence of hallucinations of some other sensory sphere in the absence of auditory hallucinations is strongly suggestive of organicity. Illusions (described below in this section), unlike hallucinations, do have a physical basis in reality, albeit distorted. Types of hallucinations include the following:

Auditory   The perception of sound or voice, ranging from an indistinct buzzing to a conversation loud enough to preclude attention to real sounds.

Autoscopic   A rare type of visual hallucination in which the patient sees a vision of himself.

Cenesthetic   Peculiar and physiologically implausible visceral sensations, such as burning in the brain.

Command   A voice is heard instructing one's behavior. Patients will sometimes find these commands irresistible, and may act accordingly, sometimes with negative consequences.

Derogatory The voice or voices in this type of auditory hallucination are insulting, criticizing, or threatening.

Formication A tactile perception of insects crawling over one's skin.

Gustatory A sensation of taste, usually unpleasant, without an actual stimulus. Generally associated with neurologic disorders.

Kinesthetic A sensation of movement in a body part that is not actually moving. May involve phantom limb (see below).

Olfactory An odor is smelled in the absence of a physical stimulus. Examples include burnt rubber, feces, and earth.

Phantom limb Perceived sensation from an amputated extremity including that it is still attached. This is not indicative of psychopathology, as it is a product of information/percepts stored in the brain from the limb that is no longer there.

Somatic Can refer to any of a variety of physical experiences, including a "rising feeling" which starts deep in the abdomen and moves into the chest or throat (a common aura of partial complex seizures). It may be difficult to distinguish from somatic delusions in psychotic individuals. For example, it is easier to label "snakes in my heart" as delusional than it is to label the concomitant "aching in my chest" as hallucinatory.

Tactile Something is felt on the skin in the absence of an actual physical stimulus. Patients may pick at themselves or think that their skin is being infested with ants (formication). Also called *haptic hallucination*.

Visual Something is seen without a physical stimulus. These may be simple, such as seeing elemental colors, a pattern, or flashing lights; or complex, such as seeing an approaching person.

Illusion An illusion is a distortion or misperception of something that is not actually present. It can be a misperception of an actual object, sound, or other sensory stimulus, most commonly in the visual realm. For example, the shadows of curtains may be misperceived as a dog. Illusions also occur in the absence of psychopathology, especially during fatigue or sleep-deprivation.

Jamais vu Less common than déjà vu, jamais vu is the feeling of unfamiliarity in a situation or environment that is actually familiar. It can occur in normal persons or in temporal lobe dysfunction.

Loose associations The loss of the normal connectedness in the subject matter of speech. In the thoughts and conversational speech of healthy individuals, sentences and ideas flow logically; during transitions between ideas, the connections are readily apparent and are related to the topic being discussed. With loose associations, the topic may suddenly shift gears, and the commonality of content or meaning may be only "loosely" apparent, with transitions based on rhymes, homonyms, or idiosyncratic mental connections. Descriptors of the connectedness of speech listed in order of increasing abnormality are normal associations; circumstantiality; tangential associations; flight of ideas; loose associations; and word salad or incoherence. Loosening of associations occurs in the context of thought disorder, most often in schizophrenia.

Magical thinking   Illogical ideas that are developmentally primitive and ascribe an unrealistic (magical) outcome or powers to an event or idea. This phenomenon is normal in children; for example, youngsters will avoid stepping on the cracks in sidewalks because it may "break their mothers' backs." It also occurs in patients with obsessive-compulsive disorder.

Mood-congruent delusion   The general tone of the delusion matches the mood: that is, grandiose and persecutory delusions in mania; and nihilistic, somatic, guilty, or persecutory delusions in depression. Other types of delusions occurring in the context of affective disorders are termed mood-incongruent. Mood-incongruent delusions may be striking; for example, a depressed person may believe that he or she is fabulously wealthy. More often the term is applied to delusions that are not closely associated with depression or mania, such as thought insertion (see Schneiderian symptoms).

Neologisms   The use of novel vocabulary, made up by the patient but not recognized by the patient as new or nonsense words. For example, "personitations" for medication side effects.

Obsessions   A consistent and persistent unwanted thought that intrudes into consciousness despite efforts to suppress it. In contrast to the situation in delusions, the patient recognizes that the thought is unrealistic. Examples of obsessions include a thought that a patient has murdered his child, a patient's hands are covered with germs, she will win the lottery, or he has left the stove on or left the door open. Sometimes the term *obsessive* is more loosely used to describe perfectionistic individuals, or anyone that worries a great deal about minor details.

Overvalued idea   An illogical or false idea that is held relatively firmly, though not quite with delusional intensity. This term is in fact useful for describing near delusions; for example, the person who is concerned that he is being poisoned acknowledges that he may be wrong and seems to accept assurances that the food is okay, yet carefully inspects it before eating.

Paranoia   Unrealistic suspiciousness and guardedness, not necessarily of delusional proportions, sometimes accompanied by grandiosity. When specific delusions are held, they should be specified (see paranoid delusion, persecutory delusion, and grandiose delusion).

Perseveration The illogical and seemingly uncontrollable repetition of an idea, phrase, or action, usually out of context and in a mechanical fashion. Distinguish from preoccupation, which is a logical and conceptually based tendency to return to the same topic or theme.

Phobia A disproportionate fear of a particular object or situation. This fear is generally recognized by the patient as irrational, yet is nonetheless disabling; and often active steps are taken to avoid the phobic situation. Major types are social phobia, the fear of being in a public situation or of being scrutinized and/or ridiculed by others, agoraphobia, the fear of open spaces (the *agora* was the old Greek marketplace), and simple phobias, such as those in this list:

Acrophobia Fear of heights

Claustrophobia Fear of closed spaces

Hemophobia Fear of blood

Homophobia Fear of homosexuals

Xenophobia Fear of strangers

Phobia may be accompanied by symptoms of autonomic hyperactivity (rapid heart rate, palpitations, rapid breathing, sweating, nausea).

Poverty of speech Little meaningful information is contained in the patient's conversation. Most commonly, this is manifested by the absence or near absence of spontaneous comment, and the response to questions with terse or one-word answers, even when elaboration is obviously in order. Alternatively, the amount of speech may be normal or even increased, yet be impoverished in content. Such speech is vague, repetitious, and circumstantial. The term poverty of thought is equivalent to poverty of speech; some use the term *poverty of content of speech* to refer specifically to cases in which speech is normal in amount but provides little information. It is considered a disorder of thought and not of language.

Preoccupation A term used to describe a topic or recurrent theme that is unduly prominent in the patient's thoughts and conversation, even when other topics are raised. Preoccupations vary in severity, from the focused enthusiasm that hobbyists may exhibit about stamps, coins, hunting, cars, or baseball teams, to having an overly focused interest in only one subject, to the exclusion of other thoughts and activities (*monomania*). Common subjects of preoccupation include health concerns, physical appearance, finances, romance, and sex.

Projection Attributing one's own thoughts, intentions, feelings, or actions to another (see Chapter 7). This is regarded as the defense mechanism responsible for paranoia, in which patients attribute hostile intent to those around them.

Psychosis   A severe mental disturbance in which thinking is disconnected from external reality; psychotic patients have a diminished ability to perceive and accept reality. Manifestations of disordered thoughts include unreal perceptions (e.g., hallucinations) and unreal beliefs (e.g., delusions). Psychosis also encompasses bizarre behavior or gross disorganization of speech that occurs without recognition by the patient that anything is amiss. Hallucinations, delusions, loose associations, and grossly disturbed behaviors are all fairly dramatic symptoms and are broadly accepted as being symptoms of psychosis; these are all referred to as *positive* psychotic symptoms. There are also *negative* psychotic symptoms, which have been largely studied in schizophrenia. Negative symptoms are defects of personality or activity that, while not considered to be proof of psychosis in themselves, often accompany psychotic conditions. These symptoms include blunting of affect (see Chapter 3); impoverished, rigid, or concrete thinking (see Chapter 6); and very poor social functioning and motivation (apathy). *Primary process thinking* is prominent in psychosis; it is symbolic and illogical thinking that is thought to occur normally in early childhood, but is relegated mostly to dreams and the unconscious as the mind develops and secondary process (more logical) thinking predominates.

Psychosis is an important but broad term; it is not a diagnostic category but, rather, a constellation of symptoms that describe a state of mentation. A number of disorders, including schizophrenia, mood disorders, and neurologic disorders, can include psychosis as part of their symptom complexes.

Racing thoughts   The subjective experience of thoughts moving very quickly from topic to topic. Racing thoughts are reported most often by patients with mania, hypomania, anxiety, hyperthyroidism, and drug intoxication (as with amphetamines).

Reduplicative paramnesia   Also known as *delusional misidentification*. The fixed delusion that one is located elsewhere, such as at home rather than a hospital (reduplicative paramnesia for place), or, the fixed belief that an imposter, often malevolent, has been substituted for one or more persons with whom the patient interacts (reduplicative paramnesia for person or *Capgras' syndrome*).

Referential thinking   The incorrect ascription of special, individualized meaning to neutral stimuli. Such thoughts are called *ideas of reference* and, unless they are very mild, can also be termed *delusions of reference*. Referential thinking often involves inappropriately personalizing information from books, television, movies, radio, or newspapers. For example, the patient may think that a television program has special meaning for him or that a newspaper article about an unrelated issue actually refers to him.

Rumination   The persistent mulling over of an unpleasant theme or thought, the way a cow ruminates its cud. Rumination is unproductive and does not reach resolution, but may be time-consuming and tends to be negative, unenjoyable, and frequently contains metaphysical, philosophic, or self-criticizing themes. Rumination is somewhat related to preoccupation but may be less narrowly focused; if the thoughts are identified by the patient as trivial or unwanted, they may be termed *ruminative obsessions*. Although rumination is not necessarily indicative of a mental illness, it occurs commonly in major depression and obsessive-compulsive disorder.

Schneiderian symptom   Any of a group of psychotic symptoms described by Austrian psychiatrist Kurt Schneider and identified as pathognomonic for schizophrenia, although subsequent research has demonstrated that these symptoms can be seen in other psychotic conditions. Among other things, Schneider's list of symptoms includes (1) hallucinations of one's own thoughts spoken aloud (*thought echo*, e.g., "I think of something and the next thing I know, I hear it"); (2) hallucinatory voices carrying on running commentary about the patient or dialogue with each other; (3) *delusional perception* (this has extreme elements of referential or magical thinking; novel, often self-referential delusions triggered by perceptual experiences, e.g., concluding that seeing a bird in a tree "means that I will be made king"); (4) feeling that drives or actions are controlled by others; (5) *thought broadcasting*, the delusional conviction that others can hear or read one's thoughts; (6) *thought insertion*, the delusional conviction that a thought is not one's own, but has been placed in one's mind by someone or something else; and (7) *thought withdrawal*, the delusional conviction that thoughts are being removed or erased from one's mind by someone or something else.

Suicidal ideation   Thoughts about killing oneself. Suicidal ideation ranges from having specific plans to kill oneself, to passive feelings or ideation, such as "I wish I were dead." It is a serious and potentially dangerous sign, as it can lead to attempted suicide. It is associated with a number of psychiatric conditions, including grief, depression, schizophrenia, anxiety, personality disorders, and substance abuse.

Suspiciousness   A mild form of paranoia; distrustfulness; vigilance for malfeasance, criticism, or aggression in others; it may be manifest in the interview setting as guardedness (see above), wariness, litigiousness, and/or lack of cooperation. Suspicious people may perceive danger or a plot without substantial evidence, and it is common in paranoid personality disorder, delusional (paranoid) disorder, and paranoid schizophrenia. However, suspiciousness does not necessarily imply psychosis.

Tangentiality   A disturbance in the associations of thinking and conversation in which the person changes the topic from the focus of the interview and follows another topic of conversation. It is named after the geometric concept of a line that touches the edge of a circle and then veers off to infinity on its own course. Tangential speech is fluent, grammatical, and logically connected, but the content will veer from the original topic into one or more different topic areas without ever returning to the topic at hand. Tangentiality is a much less severe disruption of the structure of thought than is loose association.

Thought content   The topics, ideas, or issues that the patient has on his or her mind that are cogitated over and comprise the train of thought. Normal thought content may be centered on such topics as which college to attend, a strategy for a presentation at work, or plans for an upcoming wedding. Abnormalities of thought content include delusions, magical thinking, preoccupations, ruminations, overvalued ideas, obsessions, and homicidal or suicidal ideation.

Thought disorder   A generic term that encompasses abnormalities of the content or form of thought and abnormal perceptions. This is not in itself a diagnosis and would be considered by many to be roughly equivalent to the term *psychosis*.

Thought process   The way in which thoughts flow, are connected to one another, and are expressed to the listener. Important abnormalities of thought process include loosening of associations, incoherence, word salad, flight of ideas, tangentiality, circumstantiality, blocking, clang associations, and neologisms, all of which reflect an aberrant structure of thought and disrupt normal communication. Disorders of thought process occur independently of disorders of language (see Chapter 4).

Word salad   An extreme and rare form of loosening of associations. Speech consists of a series of unconnected words and neologisms. The speech sounds fluent, but the content is incoherent. Word salad occurs mostly in schizophrenics. It resembles severe fluent aphasia (see Chapter 4), but can be differentiated by the lack of an identifiable gross brain lesion in the language areas.

References

Asaad, G., and Shapiro, B. Hallucinations: Theoretical and clinical overview. *American Journal of Psychiatry* 143: 1088–97, 1986.

Berson, R. J. Capgras' syndrome. *American Journal of Psychiatry* 140: 969–78, 1983.

Campbell, R. J. *Psychiatric Dictionary*, 6th edition. New York: Oxford University Press, 1989.

Cutting, J. *The Right Cerebral Hemisphere and Psychiatric Disorders.* New York: Oxford University Press, 1990.

Diagnostic and Statistical Manual of Mental Disorders, (Third Edition Revised.) *DSM-III-R.* Washington, D.C.: American Psychiatric Press, 1987.

Fleminger, S. Seeing is believing: The role of preconscious perceptual processing in delusional misidentification. *British Journal of Psychiatry* 160: 293–303, 1992.

Kaplan, H. I., and Sadock, B. J. *The Comprehensive Textbook of Psychiatry*, 5th edition. Baltimore: Williams and Wilkins, 1989.

Kaufman, D. M., and Solomon, S. Migraine visual auras. *General Hospital Psychiatry* 14: 162–170, 1992.

Lishman, W. A. *Organic Psychiatry: The Psychological Consequences of Cerebral Disorder*, 2nd edition. Oxford: Blackwell Scientific Publications, 1987.

Nicholi, A. M. (ed.). *The New Harvard Guide to Psychiatry.* Cambridge, Mass.: The Belknap Press of Harvard University Press, 1988.

6 | Cognition

Cognition is the ability to know and think, using intellect, logic, reasoning, memory, and all of the higher cortical functions. Intact cognition allows humans to appreciate their inner and outer worlds, and to interact with others and negotiate daily life. Thus, appropriate communication and comprehension depend not only on speech and language abilities (Chapter 4) and the absence of a thought disorder (Chapter 5), but also on other brain functions that relate to cognition and intellect. These functions should be indirectly and directly assessed during the MSE interview. In contrast to the other portions of the MSE, cognition is tested in a structured fashion. Specific assessment of a variety of cognitive functions should be completed during patient examination.

In many cases, it is useful to administer one of any number of standardized screening cognitive tests so that the patient's performance can be compared to normative data from a larger population of persons. The use of standardized tests allows a comparison to the patient's performance at a different time or when tested by a different examiner. Test scores can be recorded in the chart and graphed over time. Standardized tests range from cognitive screening tests to be used at the bedside or in the office to formal neuropsychologic testing. Screening tests can be administered in a brief period and are usually comprised of a small number of items that assess different cognitive and language abilities. One of the most widely used screening tests is the Mini-Mental state exam (see Folstein, Folstein, and McHugh, 1975), which superficially assesses a variety of cognitive functions. Screening tests can then be supplemented with more sensitive tests of specific areas of cognition.

Regardless of whether the examiner makes use of published standardized tests, or prefers to develop his or her own battery, it is important to administer the cognitive tests in a standardized fashion. The consistent use of a standard approach permits the conclusion that differences in test scores are the result of patient performance rather than the result of variations in the test or its administration.

Intellectual and cognitive abilities are related to genetics, education, and the health of the brain. Many disorders affecting the central nervous system can cause deficits in attention, memory, visuospatial ability, abstraction, and other cognitive functions. These include delirium, stroke, tumor, radiation necrosis, multiple sclerosis, Huntington's disease, parkinsonism, Alzheimer's disease, head trauma, chronic alcoholism, infections, mental retardation, and learning disabilities, to name a few. It is important to assess brain function so that diagnoses such as delirium, dementia, and amnestic syndrome can be made. Some cognitive deficits are circumscribed to one or a few cognitive skills—for example, attentional or calculation ability—whereas others are diffuse, affecting multiple or most functions—for example, as in delirium and many dementias.

Intelligence is a dimension of cognitive ability, but only a gross estimate of it can be obtained during a psychiatric interview. As intelligence quotient (IQ) is a number that allows comparison of an individual to population norms, formal testing needs to be performed in order to make a firm statement about intelligence. Often the clinician relies on the patient's verbal abilities expressed during the interview as a clue to intelligence, although this can be faulty as it does not take into account nonverbal aspects of intelligence. One might assume that the patient is of at least average intelligence (defined as an IQ of 100) if he or she graduated from college; the converse is not true, however. Highly intelligent people are distributed throughout all types of jobs and all walks of life.

The relationship between intelligence and cognition is not clear. In the presence of certain cognitive deficits (e.g., amnestic syndrome), intelligence may be reported to be unimpaired. Yet if one has several cognitive deficits, intelligence testing may not be possible.

Cognitive status affects the validity of the patient's history. It is important to be aware of possible cognitive impairment early in the interview. When it is suspected, some testing should be done immediately to determine whether the patient is capable of giving a coherent history. If the patient is unable to do so, the quality of information gathered during the interview is obviously of questionable value. There are certain clues that alert the examiner to this possibility. Risk factors for cognitive dysfunction include advanced age, head trauma, medical and neurologic illnesses that affect the brain, drugs that have central nervous system side effects either alone or in combination with other medications, drug and alcohol abuse, fever, and infection, among other concerns. If there is any cognitive impairment, the type and extent need to be determined by the use of specific tests during the interview. Whenever there is suspicion of cognitive impairment, family members, neighbors, landlords, friends, doctors, or other persons who know the patient may also need to be contacted to gather relevant facts about the patient.

If significant cognitive impairment exists, the patient may not be fully competent to accept or refuse medical or psychiatric treatment. Often a family member becomes involved formally or informally to help provide consent for the patient's continued evaluation and/or treatment. Obtaining power of attorney can be helpful, particularly when a deteriorating process such as dementia is detected early enough to allow the patient to assign power before becoming completely incompetent. In extreme cases, temporary or permanent guardianship proceedings need to be pursued through legal channels, particularly if any invasive treatments or tests are being recommended. In the event of an emergency, lifesaving medical or psychiatric evaluation and treatment can usually be started without complicated legal proceedings, which may dangerously delay needed interventions. Guidelines and policies vary from hospital to hospital, and from state to state, as to how the questionably competent patient should be handled. If guardianship proceedings are being pursued, screening cognitive tests may need to be supplemented by more formal neuropsychologic testing and by neurodiagnostic tests. Competency involves not only intact cognition as a basic condition, but also an ability to comprehend the risks/benefits and consequences of an intervention. A complete discussion of competency is beyond the scope of this text, and the reader is referred to other texts on the subject (Appelbaum and Roth, 1981; Culver and Gert, 1982; Roth, Meisel, and Lidz, 1977).

Depending on the specific tests used, and the results of the combinations of those tests, an attempt at neuroanatomic localization of abnormalities can be made. Certain areas of the cortex and subcortical areas, including the brainstem, are involved in memory, attention, executive cognitive functions, calculating ability, and so on (see Figure 6–1). In this chapter, to the extent that we understand it, localization will be mentioned for each cognitive function.

Special procedures may be applied to children and to elderly patients in the evaluation of cognition. Because of the rapidly developing intellectual and perceptual abilities of children, special tests are required for each developmental

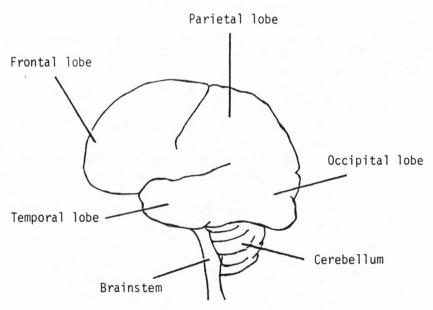

FIGURE 6–1 Major areas of the brain (lateral view), to be used for reference during discussions from text.

stage. Infants and preverbal children need to be tested more indirectly. Children cannot be expected to perform as well as adults or teenagers in some cognitive domains, because their brains have not yet fully developed. For example, children tend to be concrete in their thinking until around puberty, when most become capable of abstract thought. Aside from some general comments, it is beyond the scope of this book to include the many different specific developmental tests used for children, and the reader is referred to texts on developmental pediatrics, child psychiatry, and child neurology for more information.

The elderly tend to retain verbal skills better than so-called performance skills, such as visuomotor tasks and speed of performance. Geriatric patients have particular difficulty with timed tasks, although they may perform them accurately if they are allowed more time than one might allow a younger person. Unfortunately, there are few cognitive tests that have normative values derived exclusively from and for older persons. Thus, some special consideration may be needed when interpreting test results of geriatric patients, as the normative values obtained from younger populations may not be entirely applicable.

Application

General Comments

The cognitive portion of the MSE should be performed to some extent in any interview with a patient, and more formally during an initial evaluation or during follow-up of a patient known to be vulnerable to cognitive defects. Even without direct questioning, it is possible to obtain some cognitive information during the course of routine history-taking. For example, if a patient remembered the time, date, and location of the appointment correctly and without help from others, it is likely that orientation and prospective memory are mostly intact. If patients do not know their age, address, number of years married, ages of their children, or demographic information, then cognitive impairment is present. In the event that the patient does not know the current year, the examiner could ask the patient's year of birth and age, and say, "If you were born in 1918 and you are 75 years old, then what year does that make it now?" By doing so, one tests calculation and abstraction abilities. One might weave into the general line of questioning some tests of long-term memory of which the examiner also has knowledge and can validate the response. For example, "What did you have for breakfast?" or "Do you remember the name of that car dealer down the street where you bought your Volkswagen two years ago?" Thus, one can indirectly assess some aspects of cognitive function without performing a separate examination. Indirect questioning is particularly relevant when the patient has a dementia, since such persons often get defensive and hostile when their cognitive decline is made obvious, and they may refuse to cooperate with formal testing.

In some other situations, the examiner may feel confident from indirectly obtained information about cognition from the interview that the patient does not have cognitive impairment, without using formal testing; in this case, one would write in the chart under Cognition, "grossly intact."

It is very difficult to assess the cognition of a person who has language deficits (see Chapter 4). It is worse when the aphasia involves comprehension, as in Wernicke's aphasia. In such a case, the examiner should first try to bypass verbal comprehensive or expressive language deficits to assess cognition. Gestures and mimicry can be used to describe tasks. Designs or objects can be used to test visual memory. Jigsaw puzzles can be used to assess problem-solving skills. Attention span can be assessed by pointing to a series of written numbers. Referral to a neuropsychologist for further testing may also be useful.

Sometimes it seems awkward to ask a patient to perform cognitive tasks. The patient may appear quite intelligent and intact, and it may feel embarrassing to ask seemingly simple questions. Or, a demented elderly patient may become irritable and hostile when asked to perform cognitive tasks because the patient is aware of his or her deficits and is acting defensively. One should avoid prefacing the testing by saying "These are easy questions," because the person may be more impaired than is at first evident and then may feel worse for failing allegedly easy questions. Instead, the examiner should start with a comment like "I am going to ask you some questions which I ask all of my patients. This is to test your concentration and memory. Have you noticed any problems with getting distracted or forgetting things?" One should be prepared and have pencil and unlined white paper available, as well as the forms for whichever standardized tests are being used. One should ascertain that the patient can comprehend, read, and write before proceeding with tests of attention, memory, calculations, and so on (see Chapter 4 for language tests). A quiet room and a comfortable setting should be reserved for the patient, so that he or she can perform cognitive testing without interruption. Noise from external sources (phone calls, paging systems, etc.) should be kept to a minimum. In addition to external distractions, alterations in motivation and mood can also affect performance on cognitive testing.

The overall *level of consciousness* should be noted. This ranges from normal alertness and awareness to drowsiness, delirium, stupor, or coma (see Chapter 2). Obviously, a person in coma cannot perform a cognitive examination. However, documentation of cognitive deficits can be important in order to diagnose delirium. In delirium, the level of consciousness may wax and wane, with periods (minutes to hours) of relative lucidity as well as periods of overt confusion or sleepiness.

Table 6.1. Cognitive testing sequence

---

1. Orientation to person, place, and time
2. Attention and concentration
3. Registration and short-term memory
   (verbal and nonverbal)
4. Long-term memory (verbal and nonverbal)
5. Constructional and visuospatial ability
6. Abstraction and conceptualization

Table 6–1 lists a typical sequence for cognitive examination during the MSE. This sequence is followed in the sections below.

Orientation

Orientation to person, place, and time is a basic cognitive function. Essentially, this means that patients should know who they are, where they are, and what the time and date are. Orientation to time, place, and person assesses a type of memory function (temporal or prospective memory). When disorientation occurs, it usually proceeds with the sense of time lost first, followed by place and, lastly, person. *Orientation to time* is tested by asking the time of day, day of the week, month, day of the month, year, and season. Hospitalized patients commonly lose track of the exact day of the month, but should remain clear on the month, season, and year, and should be close on the day of the week and whether it is the beginning, middle, or end of the month. *Orientation to place* is tested by determining whether the patient knows the name of the hospital or clinic and the floor; also important are the city and state in which the interview is taking place. *Orientation to person* means to one's self, to one's family and friends, and to those in contact with the patient in the hospital or clinic. Impairment usually begins with those least well known to the patient: the nurses, doctors, therapists. Their names or functions may be forgotten, and, more commonly, they may be misidentified as hotel staff, as an old friend, or as torturers. Next, more familiar persons, like neighbors or family members, may be misidentified. And finally, the patient may no longer know his or her own identity; this is a very grave sign in a delirious patient.

Although disorientation is most commonly observed in confusional states and severe amnestic syndromes, extensive damage to the prefrontal cortex (usually bilateral) may result in disorientation. An unusual condition, called transient global amnesia, also involves temporary disorientation and memory deficits, possibly related to temporal lobe dysfunction. Moderately to severely demented persons can become disoriented. Sedation from medications, too, can interfere with orientation. Damage to the frontal lobes from trauma or surgery can also impair orientation. Psychotic patients usually retain reasonably good orientation, unless impaired by marked disorganization of thought processes or marked pre-occupation with delusions or hallucinations.

Attention and Concentration

Attention and concentration are related functions. *Attention* is the ability to focus and direct cognitive processes while in a physiologically aroused state. *Concentration* is the ability to focus and sustain attention for a period of time. Attentional deficits frequently interfere with performance in other realms of cognition. Attentional functions are mediated by a network of cortical and sub-cortical brain regions, with the brainstem reticular activating system providing arousal as a precondition to attending to specific inputs. Subcortical areas, such as the cingulate gyrus, parts of the thalamus, and the ascending noradrenergic, dopaminergic, and cholinergic brainstem pathways, act in conjunction with the prefrontal cortex and nondominant inferior parietal lobe to subserve attentional functions. Because there are varied aspects of attention, there are different areas of attention to test, including visual, auditory, and verbal. Brief bedside tests are available, as well as standardized tests for assessment of attention and concentration. Attention and concentration are related functions, although attention may still be intact while concentration is not, as, for example, in early Alzheimer's dementia. Patients who are agitated and generally distractible (see Chapter 2) during the interview are likely to have attentional deficits. Those who are anx-ious, sleep-deprived, actively psychotic, in pain, or are children with attention deficit disorder, are likely to be impaired on attentional testing, especially concentration.

Standardized tests that assess attention and concentration include the Trail-making Tests, Symbol Digit Test, Mesulam's Cancellation Tests, and Stroop Color–Word Test. These are discussed in the various sections that follow.

ATTENTION

Measurement of *digit span* is a commonly used attentional test. Digits (single numbers) are recited to the patient in series of increasing lengths. After each series, the patient is asked to repeat it aloud. Writing is not allowed. For exam-ple, the examiner should say, "I want you to repeat the following numbers after I say them: 5-2-9-4." Then the patient should reply, "5-2-9-4." The examiner should recite the digits in a monotone, except for the last digit which is said in a lowered pitch to indicate it is the final digit of that series. If the examiner does not speak in a monotone, the musicality used (*prosody*) may inappropriately aid the patient in repeating the digit span. Each number of a series should be recited to the patient slowly and clearly, at about one-second intervals. The intervals should remain consistent, to avoid inappropriately cluing the patient (e.g., grouping digits like phone numbers). Begin with a two-digit series, then proceed to a three-digit series, four, five, and so on, until the patient cannot perform correctly. Once the *digit span*—that is, the maximum number of digits done correctly on two consecutive trials—is established, then the patient should be asked to repeat some series backwards. The examiner should say, "1-2-3," after which the patient should say, "3-2-1." This task should first be illustrated so that the patient understands its nature. Again, the examiner should proceed from a two-digit series in upward increments until the patient makes a mistake, for determining first the forward and then the backward digit span. Usually the forward span is one to two digits higher than the backward span. Normal forward spans are 6 ± 1 digits; they remain stable intraindividually into old age. Most normal, healthy adults can perform seven digits forward (as in phone numbers) and five digits backward. In general, if the number of digits backward is more than two fewer than forward, it is abnormal and implies a problem in divided attention (i.e., attending while distracted by another mental task, as in changing the order of digit recitation). Digit span is impaired in delirious, moderately demented, and frontal/subcortical-lesioned patients, who may perform normally on the forward span, but do poorly on backward span. Left frontal-lobe dysfunction can shorten the forward digit span. Abulic patients perform slowly and may not complete this task.

Visual attention tests can also be used; they involve pictures with items, such as birds, hidden within a scene. The patient is asked to point to and count aloud each bird he or she can find in the picture.

CONCENTRATION
A simple test of concentration is to ask the patient to "count backward starting at 65 and stopping at 49." The task should be stated only once and not repeated after the counting has begun. Inattentive persons will continue counting beyond 49, or will lose track of the task during the counting. This is a good test for the elderly, in whom serial sevens (see below) may be too sensitive to the effects of normal aging.

Concentration, or sustained attention, can also be tested by asking patients to calculate *serial seven subtractions* "in their heads"—that is, without writing or other external help. Arithmetic testing can provide an assessment of impairment not only in calculation ability but also in concentration. The patient should be asked to "start at 100 and subtract 7, then keep subtracting 7 from each answer." One would expect the response to be "100-93-86-79-72-65" from a person without concentration difficulties. If the patient makes an error part way through the sequence, but then continues to subtract in intervals of seven, consider any interval of seven to be correct. The examiner should allow one point for each correct interval of seven; generally the patient should be asked to perform five subtractions. For example, a response of "100-93-85-78-71-64" would be scored as four points out of a maximum of five. Patients who have difficulty concentrating might try to think out loud—for example, "7 from 86: 6 from 86 is 80, then 1 from 80 is 79." Or they might try to use their fingers (discourage this). Or they might lose track of the task, or have long pauses between numbers. These are all indicative of some degree of difficulty in concentrating, even if the calculations are correct. In addition to using serial sevens from 100, one could use serial sevens from 101 or serial 13's from 100. For patients who are having trouble with the arithmetic, substitute serial three subtractions from 20, or serial additions from one in intervals of three. As a baseline, one should ascertain that the patient can perform simple arithmetic. Patients who have fewer than eight years of education may find serial seven subtractions too difficult. Patients older than 70 years may have difficulty with serial seven subtractions, but educational or occupational background (e.g., a retired accountant) should be taken into account when assessing this difficulty. Easier calculations or nonmathematical tasks, such as spelling a word backward, can be substituted. Of course, inability to perform serial sevens suggests attentional impairment in a well-educated patient, even if he or she can accurately perform easier tasks.

On a popular screening test, the Mini-Mental State Exam, spelling the word "WORLD" backward is used as an alternative to serial sevens. In this case, each letter should be scored as a point only if it is both in the correct order and in the correct position. Thus, "DLROW" is correct for five points, whereas "DLOW" is scored only two points. The word "EARTH" can also be used. Another simpler test of concentration is to recite the days of the week or months of the year backward.

Memory

Our brains store a virtual library of information and past experiences. The process of learning involves registering information, storing it, and later retrieving it from memory (see Fig. 6–2). Some memories are temporary, whereas others become more permanent. While there is controversy in the field regarding terminology and neuroanatomy of memory, we have chosen to use Squire's (1986) descriptions for this chapter.

Registration is the capacity for immediate recall of new learning; it lasts only a few seconds. It is variously considered to precede memory or to be the initial component of short-term memory.

There are two major types of memory: short-term and long-term memory. *Short-term memory* precedes the consolidation of long-term memories (see Figure 6–2) and occurs successfully only if attention to and registration of information precede it. Short-term memory is temporary, lasting from seconds to a few minutes; this information can be used immediately in decision making and/or it passes into long-term memory. Short-term memory is limited in capacity and

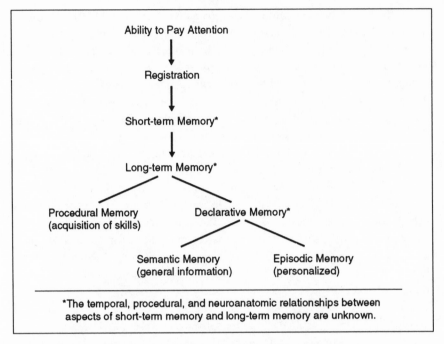

FIGURE 6-2   Schematic of types of memory.

can be saturated; in contrast, there are no evident limits to the storage capacity of long-term memory.

There are two types of *long-term memory:* procedural and declarative. *Procedural memory* involves remembering how to perform a set of skills, like driving, skiing, swimming, or riding a bicycle. After initial practice and mastery of these perceptual–motor skills, procedural memories become implicit—that is, not in conscious awareness. Procedural memory remains intact in most amnestic patients, both for previously learned skills and for learning new skills. Procedural memory is phylogenetically old and is not affected by dysfunction of the temporal lobe–diencephalic areas known to be important for other types of long-term memory. Procedural memory is typically not assessed in the MSE.

Declarative memory, which is affected in amnestic patients, involves data or facts that can be verbal or nonverbal (e.g., images or sounds), as opposed to skills or procedures. It is explicit in that remembered information should be retrievable into conscious awareness, unless there is damage to the brain areas involved in the storage and/or retrieval of these memories (i.e., amnestic syndrome) or there is a psychologic defense mechanism interfering with their retrieval (e.g., repression, dissociation, or denial; see Chapter 7). Declarative memories are phylogenetically more recent and are located in the medial temporal lobe, hippocampus, diencephalon, and ventromedial frontal lobe areas. Declarative memory continues to be consolidated over time and can also decay over time (gradual forgetting). It has been hypothesized that the various types of short-term memory (verbal, visual, auditory) are located in the same brain areas as their associated long-term memory storage sites with which they interact. The medial temporal region is particularly important during learning and for consolidation of long-term declarative memory. Eventual retrieval of information from long-term memory involves coordination between the medial temporal area and various storage sites in the cortex.

Retrograde amnesia refers to a loss of long-term memories that were consolidated just prior to the insult or event that produced the amnesia (e.g., car accident or stroke), whereas *anterograde amnesia* refers to the time period subsequent to the incident—that is, the inability to learn, store, and retrieve new information as part of long-term memory. For example, head trauma patients often have some degree of retrograde amnesia, usually for hours or days just prior to the accident, as well as anterograde amnesia for information about the accident and from a period after the trauma that usually lasts for hours or days. In some cases anterograde amnesia extends indefinitely, that is, it becomes an amnestic syndrome.

Patients with Korsakoff's amnesia have diencephalic dysfunction with profound anterograde long-term memory deficits and variable retrograde amnesia (often remote memories are intact), but with preservation of registration and short-term memory. Thus, they are able to recall newly presented information after a few seconds or minutes, but do not remember it hours or days later. Bilateral paramedian thalamic lesions or third ventricle tumors cause severe anterograde amnesia for long-term memory. Dominant temporal lobe lesions predominantly affect verbal memory, whereas nondominant temporal lobe lesions affect visual memory. Bilateral temporal lobe lesions cause more severe amnesia than unilateral lesions and greatly impair new learning (anterograde memory); attention span is normal, however, as is short-term memory, and recent long-term memory is often more impaired than very remote long-term memory (retrograde amnesias). Viral encephalitis (commonly Herpes), infarctions due to posterior cerebral artery compromise, and hypoxia (e.g., cardiac arrest or carbon monoxide poisoning) can cause bitemporal lesions and amnesia.

Pseudodementia is a term used in describing patients whose memory deficits are presumably due to physiologic perturbations associated with a psychiatric disturbance, rather than to structural brain damage. Pseudodemented patients show a pattern of "spotty" deficits and inconsistent performance on most memory testing, related to their attentional deficits and inconsistent motivation. Truly demented patients have difficulty with long-term memory, usually more with recent than with remote information, until later in the disease when both are impaired.

Patients with frontal lobe damage have deficits in *temporal memory* or *prospec-*

tive memory, which is remembering to remember. This is not a consequence of a true amnesia, but is related to the inability to shift mental sets from one topic to another in order to focus on newly presented information and then remember it, and to deficits in planning and organization abilities (i.e., what to do tomorrow and the day after). These so-called temporal memory deficits also affect orientation (see above). With sufficient focusing and rehearsal, frontal lobe-lesioned patients can remember information—once the volitional/motivational impairments are overcome.

REGISTRATION

To learn and remember, one must first pay attention (see Table 6–2). Assuming that attentional abilities are intact, memory can be tested. Before assessing memory, the examiner should ensure that registration of the information has occurred. The examiner should assess registration via *immediate recall* (within seconds) of the material presented to the patient. For example, the patient may be presented with words to remember after a delay. The examiner might say, "I am going to tell you three words which I want you to remember, and I shall ask you about them in a few minutes. The words are red, table, and coat. Please repeat them now so I shall know you heard them." If the patient can repeat them, registration has apparently occurred. If not, the examiner should repeat them and ask the patient to recite them until they are registered. The number of trials required for registration should be noted; more than two trials suggests inadequate registration. It is particularly important to ensure that registration has occurred in inattentive, poorly motivated, or depressed patients. Immediate recall is closely related to attentional ability. Patients with registration difficulties may complain of being forgetful when in actuality, rather than a true amnesia, the patient may have a registration defect.

Once attention and registration abilities have been established, tests of short-term and long-term memory can be administered. Both verbal and nonverbal material can be tested.

SHORT-TERM MEMORY

To test short-term memory, the examiner presents three or four unrelated words to be remembered after a five-minute delay. He or she checks for adequate registration, as previously described, then proceeds with other tasks of the MSE. After five minutes, the patient is asked to state the words that were requested. One point is scored for each correctly remembered word in this short-term recall test (e.g., "recall is 2/3 words after 5 minutes"). Then, to assess further the severity of any recent memory deficit, the patient is cued for any missing words using a category: If the forgotten word is "brown," mention that "it's a color"; if the forgotten word is "bird," mention that "it's something that flies." The examiner should not score any points for a word recalled by category cuing, but record that cuing was helpful. If category cues do not help, then the examiner should give several possible words, including the correct one, from which the patient can choose. If the patient recognizes the forgotten word from this multiple choice list, no points are scored, but the performance in the MSE is noted.

Another test of short-term memory is to read a paragraph-long vignette aloud. The examiner should preface it by explaining to the patient that he or she will be expected to retell the story from memory. When the patient retells the story, the examiner counts the number of important words or phrases remembered. An example might be:

George/ is a T.V./ news reporter./ He was covering an earthquake/ in Los Angeles./ He interviewed/ a woman,/ named Carol,/ whose car/ was parked on a street/ which caved in/ during the tremors./ The car/ disappeared/ into the earth./

In each sentence the different notable phrases to be recalled are separated by brackets to illustrate the 15 different ideas expressed. Remembering at least 8 of them would be a normal performance; the recall does not need to be verbatim, but should include the important words. Of course, examiners can make up their own vignettes.

Verbal short-term memory can be further tested using a word-list learning task. The patient is asked to remember two different types of word lists, each consisting of 15 words: The first list is comprised of words related by categories; the other contains unrelated words. Before each trial, the patient is instructed to remember as many words as possible, but that the order of recall does not matter (i.e., within each type of list). Each list is tested separately, beginning with the related (categorized) list, with two trials for each list. Each word is read aloud by the examiner at a rate of about one per second, then immediately repeated by the patient. This is done twice (read aloud by the examiner in a different order for the second trial) to give the patient two chances to learn the word list. After each trial the patient is asked to recite as many of the words as possible, even if the words recalled after the second trial include some of those recited for that list's first trial. The patient is allowed one minute to recite recalled items after each trial, and one point is scored for each word recalled; a total score for each word list consists of the sum of trial one points plus trial two points. The related list is scored separately from the unrelated list. Examples of lists of related and unrelated words follow:

List A	List B
Dog	Vacuum
Chicken	Truck
Horse	Movie

Cat	Conference
Elephant	Envelope
Book	Fire
Magazine	Election
Newspaper	Moon
Pamphlet	Refrigerator
File	Shovel
Knife	House
Dish	Lemonade
Pan	Town
Spatula	Wallet
Grill	Lamp

List A is easier to recall because the words are associated into categories (animals, reading items, and kitchen items). It requires more effort to recall List B. Normal persons will remember a total of about 16 words from the two trials on each list with similar performances for the related and unrelated lists. Amnestic syndrome patients do not group words of a category together in order to enhance recall, so will perform similarly on both lists. A patient with depression-induced pseudodementia will do fairly well on the related list, but more poorly on the unrelated list, because of reduced motivation and impaired attention to the more challenging task. A truly demented person will do poorly with both lists. Thus, word list recall may help to distinguish normal from pseudodemented from demented persons. If the words from each list are again requested for recall following a 20-minute delay (without the list being reread), then long-term verbal memory can be assessed.

It is also important to assess nonverbal short-term memory. *Visual short-term memory* can be tested by showing patients a picture of six simple designs for five seconds and then having them draw what they remember. Because drawing is involved, a visual or visuospatial deficit might interfere with the ability to test memory. To test for such a confound, a trial at simply copying designs can follow the failed recall trial, to detect a visuospatial constructional impairment. Alternatively, visual memory testing can involve recognition of shapes or designs instead of actually having patients draw them. After a period of studying several designs, patients are asked to identify them from among a larger selection of similar designs. Figure 6–3 shows three figures that can be used in testing nonverbal memory, with these same figures distributed among other designs for use in recognition recall.

To test *auditory short-term memory*, the examiner taps a pattern of loud and soft sounds and asks the patient to repeat the pattern(s). The examiner should start with simple patterns and progress to more complicated ones.

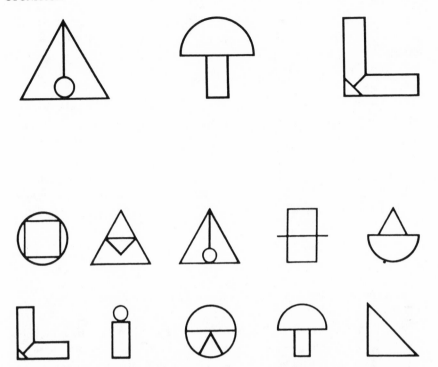

FIGURE 6–3   Designs from Mesulam's Three Shapes Test that can be used to test visual memory and recognition recall following a delay. (Reproduced from Mesulam, M-M. *Principles of Behavioral Neurology.* Philadelphia: F. A. Davis, 1985, by permission of F. A. Davis, publishers.)

LONG-TERM MEMORY

Long-term memory can be either recent or remote, depending on the time period in question. Remote memories are those from many years ago, such as events from childhood. Both the episodic and semantic subtypes of declarative long-term memory can be assessed.

Episodic memory is time-tagged, personalized, and experiential knowledge. The patient is asked to describe important personal events, such as a wedding, entering college, past medical history, and so on, and to identify when these events happened. The examiner should verify from other sources the data gathered from episodic memory testing; family, neighbors, or old medical charts can help. One can informally gather episodic information while eliciting the patient's past medical and psychiatric history during the interview. The examiner should be wary of *confabulation*; a patient with memory deficits may go on and on with interesting stories that have no basis in fact. Particularly grandiose or unbelievable stories may indicate *spontaneous confabulation*. For example, a patient hospitalized for frontal lobe damage may spontaneously confabulate that she is a nurse and will be leaving the hospital unit at 3:30 P.M. with the other nurses, that she had a tough day caring for patients, that she is going out to dinner and then the symphony that evening, and that she'll be on vacation tomorrow.

Semantic memory involves recall of general information that a person could reasonably be expected to have learned. For example, one can test it by asking "Who were the last five U.S. presidents?" or "When did World War II end?" or "What famous college is in Cambridge, Massachusetts?" or "Where do the Steelers play?" Minutiae and trivia are not fair to ask, however. Semantic memory can also be tested by asking the patient to list orally as many things as possible in one minute that can be purchased in a grocery store. Normal persons can list at least 18 different things.

Constructional Ability

Prerequisites for *constructional ability* are intact vision, motor coordination, strength, praxis, and tactile sensation. Patients who fail construction tests may need to be tested for other disorders that could interfere with their ability to perform well, including visual deficits, writing apraxia, and visual agnosia. Vision can be screened by using an eye chart or by confrontational visual field testing. The examiner performs confrontational field testing by outstretching his or her arms about a foot in front and slightly to each side of the patient (so that they fall in the temporal hemifields), extending each index finger upward, and instructing the patient to stare straight ahead. Then one or both fingers are wiggled and the patient is asked which side moved. This is performed at three levels in space: both arms horizontal, left arm up and right arm down, and left arm down and right arm up. The patient should be able to see and identify the moving finger(s) in all fields. Next, the examiner tests writing using a pen to ensure that the patient does not have a writing apraxia.

Constructional ability and visuospatial function are essential to performing many everyday activities. They are necessary to drive, maneuver in the kitchen to cook, use a computer, vacuum a room, climb the stairs, read maps, solve mazes, and get around the environment without becoming lost. Deficits can have many consequences, and yet patients may not be able specifically to describe their disabilities in clinical terms. A patient may complain of not recognizing previously familiar faces of friends at social functions, leading to frustration and depression, or may no longer be capable of knitting or doing puzzles with the children. Testing is important to clarify the nature of the underlying deficits.

Constructing figures in two or three dimensions and solving geometric puzzles require an integration of motor and visuospatial functions. While the nondominant (right) hemisphere is particularly important for visuospatial function, both

hemispheres have a capacity for imagery and both contribute to visuoconstructional skills, albeit in different ways. The nondominant hemisphere's expertise
(especially the parietal area) is to perceive overall form or Gestalt, whereas the left
hemisphere discerns details. The approach the patient takes while drawing complex figures (see clockface and Rey–Osterrieth below) may offer clues to lateraliz-
ation of the affected brain area. Abnormalities in drawings by right hemisphere-
lesioned patients include loss of spatial relations, incorrect orientation, scattered
and fragmented components, and new lines added in an attempt to correct the
drawing. Patients with left hemisphere impairment typically draw a coherent but
simplified image without details but with a correct overall spatial orientation and
relations. Lesions to the posterior parietal areas, as in Alzheimer's dementia,
alter constructional ability. Visual agnosia, a rare condition, may make it difficult for patients to recognize things visually, although they can feel an object and
identify it. The presence of visual agnosia may confound visuospatial testing.

An easy way to assess constructional ability is to begin by having the patient
copy a three-dimensional square (block) (see Figure 6–4). The Mini-Mental

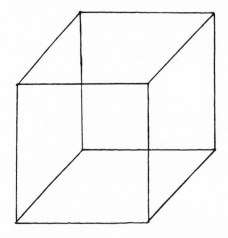

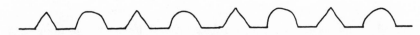

FIGURE 6–4   A cube and a repeating design, which can be used to test visuoconstructional ability.

State Exam uses intersecting pentagons to assess construction. Figure 6–5 shows this test item (upper left) and examples of actual patient attempts to copy it, all of which are impaired. If the patient cannot copy these pentagons, simpler geometric designs, like circles, triangles, or squares, can be tried. A pattern of alternating shapes (i.e., graphomotor sequences as in Figure 6–4) for the patient to copy not only tests constructional ability but also may detect motor perseveration of

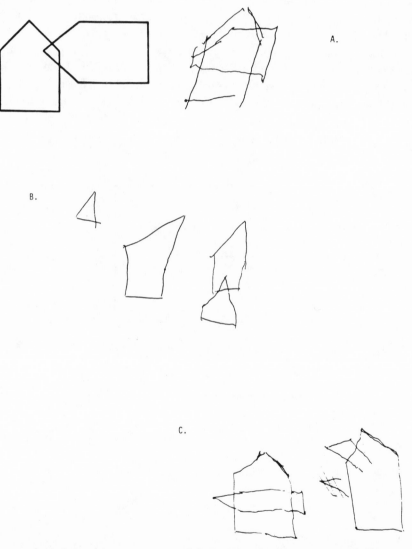

FIGURE 6–5   Intersecting pentagons and three patients' attempts to copy them. Each patient (A, B, C) had dementia, more severely in cases B and C, both of whom made two attempts at drawing.

one of the shapes. If the patient cannot copy this alternating design, the examiner should have him or her draw its simpler components, the circle and the triangle.

Clock drawing is a convenient and sensitive screening test. The examiner asks the patient to draw a clockface. The examiner chooses a time to be drawn, such as "twenty after eight" or "ten to eleven," so that the long and short hands are not perpendicular to or overlapping each other. Figure 6–6 shows examples of actual patients' clock drawings, each of which is impaired. Right-handed patients who have *anosognosia* (neglect) may ignore the left side of the drawing or squeeze most of the drawing onto the right side, as seen in example B in Figure 6–6. (Another test of neglect might be to give the patient a pair of gloves; the anosognosic patient will put only the right glove on.) Patients with visuospatial deficits will space the numbers unevenly, put them outside of the circle, or otherwise distort the clockface. The hands may not point to the correct time setting requested. Motor perseveration may impede finishing the task, with the patient becoming stuck in one area and drawing it over and over. The left hemisphere normally contributes the capacity to draw details like position of the hands and size of the numbers, whereas the right hemisphere perceives rotations or distortions of the whole shape or layout and the spatial relationship and proportionality among the components. If patients are severely impaired in drawing a clockface (as in Figure 6–6), the examiner may need to test separately the patient's ability to write numbers or to count aloud. When administered as a screening test, the clockface drawing offers valuable information; if quantification is needed, Table 6–2 describes a scoring system.

Puzzles also test constructional ability. One can use actual puzzle pieces for the patient to complete, or one can draw sections of an object on a piece of paper and ask the patient to imagine what the "whole" object would look like. Figure 6–7 shows examples from the Hooper Visual Test (Hooper, 1958), a standardized test that can be used for this purpose. The Hooper also assesses reasoning ability, because the pieces need to be imagined as a functional whole without moving the pieces. Right hemisphere and frontal lobe functions are important for performance of this task. Alternatively, one can use red-tipped matches to make geometric designs and ask the patient to replicate the designs. (When done again from memory after a delay, this tests long-term visual memory ability.) Not only is the general shape important (e.g., square), but the more subtle positioning of the red tips should be replicated by the patient. In these types of visuoconstructional tasks, drawing is not necessary.

Asking the patient to draw a map of the United States and to indicate the locations of various important cities, like New York, San Francisco, Boston, Miami, Dallas, Chicago, and San Diego, tests visuospatial function and general information (semantic memory) at the same time. The general shape of the country should be proportionate, the peninsula of Florida should be drawn, and

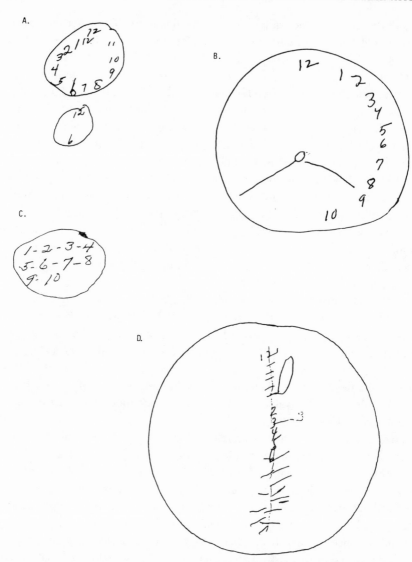

FIGURE 6–6   Four patients' attempts to draw a clockface. Patient A, who had dementia, reversed the numbers and deleted the hands. Patient B appeared to neglect the left side, except when adding the hands; she was pseudodemented and inattentive, as a result of major depression; a second attempt was done correctly, demonstrating that the apparent neglect was probably the result of poor planning. Patient C, also demented, was quite impaired, missing the proper spatial arrangement of numbers (the examiner drew the circle). Drawing D is also very impaired with an incomplete and linear arrangement of numbers and lines; this was done by the same patient three months after the drawing labeled A, when her dementia had progressed.

Table 6.2. Clockface drawing 10-point scoring system

10	Normal drawing, numbers and hands in approximately correct positions, hour hands distinctly different from minute hand and approaching correct hour number.
9	Slight errors in placement of hands or one missing number on clockface.
8	More noticeable errors in placement of hour and minute hand (off by one number); number spacing shows a gap.
7	Placement of hands significantly off course (> one number); very inappropriate spacing of numbers (e.g., all on one side).
6	Inappropriate use of clock hands (e.g., digital display or circling of numbers); crowding of numbers at one end of the clock or reversal of numbers.
5	Perseverative or otherwise inappropriate arrangement of numbers (e.g., numbers indicated by dots). Hands may be represented, but do not clearly point at a number.
4	Numbers absent, written outside of clock or in distorted sequence. Integrity of the clockface missing. Hands not clearly represented.
3	Numbers and clockface no longer connected in the drawing. Hands not recognizably present.
2	Drawing reveals some evidence of instructions received, but representation of clock is only vague; inappropriate spatial arrangement of numbers.
1	Irrelevant, uninterpretable figure or no attempt.

Source: Spreen, O., and Strauss, E. A Compendium of Neuropsychological Tests: Administration, Norms, and Commentary. New York: Oxford University Press, 1991. (Reproduced by permission.)

Hawaii and Alaska should not be forgotten. Cities and oceans should be correctly located. One should not score for quality of artwork if the general idea is there. Likewise, tremor, as from lithium treatment, may cause lines to be somewhat wiggly; this should be taken into consideration. Chorea may significantly impair drawings when visuospatial abilities may be otherwise intact. One may also use standardized drawings, such as the Rey–Osterrieth complex design (Osterrieth, 1944), which are even more challenging tests of constructional ability.

Abstraction and Conceptualization

Abstraction and higher conceptual thinking are apparently uniquely human capabilities, separating us from other animals. Higher conceptual (executive) ability includes the capacity to be aware of oneself, one's thoughts, and one's behavior. The size of our frontal lobes probably reflects these capacities. Our frontal lobes occupy about 30% of our total cerebral cortical volume, a far greater percentage than in other animals (Fuster, 1980). Brains of chimpanzees have about 17% frontal lobe, dogs about 7%, and cats about 3.5%, evincing an

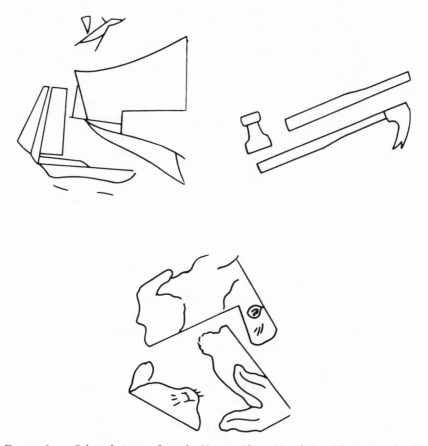

FIGURE 6–7   Selected pictures from the Hooper Object Visual Test. The patient should visualize the whole object from these dissociated parts (sailboat, hammer, and rabbit). (Reproduced from Hooper, H. E. *The Hooper Visual Organization Test: Manual.* Los Angeles: Western Psychological Services, 1958, by permission of Western Psychological Services.)

evolutionary trend toward increasing size of frontal lobes with increasing phylogenetic development (Fuster, 1980).

The frontal lobes are interconnected with many other brain areas, allowing for integration and sharing of information among areas with different primary functions. Frontal lobes are involved in attention, prospective memory (remembering to remember), conceiving and organizing for the future (temporal relationships), motivation, spontaneity, creativity, abstract thought, and ability to initiate activity. The frontal cortex is important for what are termed *executive functions*, which regulate complex and novel thinking, judgments, and behaviors. In the dominant hemisphere, the frontal lobe is also important for language (see Broca's aphasia, under Aphasias, in Chapter 4).

The prefrontal cortex is part of an interconnected cortical and subcortical network that includes association areas in the temporal and parietal lobes, limbic regions, and subcortical nuclei. Thus, deficits in executive functions can occur because of lesions or degeneration of basal cholinergic and midbrain dopaminergic nuclei, the caudate nuclei, or the medial dorsal thalamic nuclei, or because of multiple subcortical white matter lesions that disrupt corticocortical connections, or multiple cortical lesions outside the frontal lobe. Memory, attention, and visuospatial ability integrate with frontal executive ability in the production of abstract thinking and sophisticated conceptualization; deficits in any of these cognitive abilities, or in language, can affect executive functions.

Abstract thinking is the capacity to conceptualize meanings of words beyond the most literal (concrete) interpretation. This includes the ability to analyze information according to themes, to generalize according to categories, to appreciate double meanings, to make comparisons, to hypothesize, and to reason using deductive and inductive thinking. It corresponds to Piaget's "formal operations" period of cognitive development, a more advanced stage of thinking and reasoning. Abstracting ability may be affected by education, intelligence, and cultural factors, and by developmental level in children. The left hemisphere's contribution to abstract thinking is the capacity to formulate verbal concepts, using rules of hierarchy and logic; the right hemisphere's contribution is the capacity to appreciate an overall, integrated image of the spatial, emotional (e.g., humor), and practical components. Humor often involves switching mental sets between concrete and abstract interpretations of material; such switches catch the listener off-guard, leading to laughter when the leap is realized.

Concreteness may be indirectly evident during the MSE interview. If the examiner asks, "What brought you to the hospital?" an abstract answer might be, "I have been feeling depressed." A concrete answer might be, "The ambulance." Because concrete answers are not expected, they might at first seem humorous or lead the examiner to think the patient is trying to be facetious.

Assessment of the ability to identify similarities and interpret proverbs is a common approach to testing abstraction. During *similarities* comparisons, the patient is asked to conceptualize the category to which two items belong. The examiner says, "In what way are an apple and an orange alike?" The correct answer is that they are both fruit; this is an abstract answer. An answer that they both are round is concrete; that they can both be eaten is somewhat less concrete. Other similarities that are commonly used include a car and a boat (both modes of transportation), a shirt and a coat (both clothing), a table and a chair (both furniture). When asked how a dog and a tree are alike, an answer that they both have bark is literal, though almost a pun. The correct answer is that they are both living things.

Proverb interpretation is another way to test abstraction. It also measures divergent reasoning. Proverbs are intrinsically significant when generalized or abstracted, rather than in literal interpretation. Proverbs vary in their level of complexity; some persons may be able to interpret only the simpler ones. Easier proverbs include the following: "The grass is greener on the other side," "Don't count your chickens before they hatch," and "A stitch in time saves nine." Abstract interpretations of these are, respectively, "Things that seem better elsewhere are not necessarily so," "Don't be prematurely expecting something that might not happen," and "Take action today to avoid consequences or complications tomorrow." Possible concrete interpretations are, respectively, "His lawn is greener than mine," "You won't know how many chicks will be born by counting the eggs," and "Sewing prevents more rips." The following are examples of more difficult proverbs: "Rome wasn't built in a day," "People who live in glass houses shouldn't throw stones," "Loose lips sink ships," "Every cloud has a silver lining," and "A rolling stone gathers no moss."

One should begin by explaining to the patient what is meant by a *proverb*; it is a saying with a broader meaning. An example should be found that the patient may already have heard, such as "Save for a rainy day." Then one should proceed with easy proverbs for interpretation. If patients can interpret simple ones, then one should progress to harder ones. There are several possible explanations for an inability to interpret proverbs abstractly: inadequate education (less than eight years), acute psychosis, dementia, delirium, head injury, frontal lobe damage, low IQ (including mental retardation), and lack of cultural applicability of the proverb. Sometimes because interpretations of easier proverbs have been learned, patients can recite them from memory; still they cannot reason out unfamiliar ones.

Another aspect of conceptualization is the ability to switch mental sets quickly—for example, between letters and numbers (see the Trailmaking B Test in the following section), or between symbols and numbers (see Stroop Test below), or between motor tasks. Alternation between motor tasks can be tested by asking the patient to squeeze the examiner's hand whenever he or she says "green" and to relax whenever he or she says "red" (a Go–No go *paradigm*). Impulsive and prefrontal cortex-lesioned patients are particularly apt to make errors of omission, commission, and perseveration on such tasks.

Standardized Tests

The examiner may wish to supplement the informal screening for cognitive deficits done during the course of the interview with more challenging or more specific tests that are standardized. Consistent use of the same screening tests during routine cognitive examinations "standardizes" a battery across different patients. From the various screening tests already mentioned, regular administration of some from each category is recommended. The examiner should select at least one to test each cognitive function: orientation, attention and concentration (including calculation tasks), short-term memory, long-term memory, construction, and conceptualization. Sample screening batteries are listed in Table 6–3.

In addition, there are standardized test forms that either address one particular function, like attention, or incorporate a variety of tasks so that the score reflects many functions. These can be added to the screening battery to amplify the cognitive exam. Standardized tests have been administered to populations of patients and normal persons so that cutoff scores or percentile ranks are determined for use in distinguishing normal from abnormal performances. Generally these tests have been published and are available for use by the clinician, researcher, or practicing neuropsychologist. There are many different test batteries, specific for various purposes; for example, there are tests designed specifically for children, for intelligence testing, or for memory testing. The tests mentioned below are but a small sample from the standardized instruments available, but seem particularly useful for MSE testing, both for screening and for testing specific areas of cognition. Readers interested in testing preverbal or verbal children should refer to specialized texts devoted to those age groups.

Referral to a neuropsychologist for formal IQ testing may also be helpful. A commonly used IQ test is the *Wechsler Adult Intelligence Scale* (WAIS). Its information and vocabulary subtests are believed to be robust indictors of premorbid intellectual abilities. Verbal aspects of intelligence, as measured by tests like the WAIS, may remain relatively constant as a person ages; on the other hand, the so-called performance aspects of intelligence appear to be more vulnerable to the effects of aging as well as to certain psychiatric disorders such as conduct disorder, alcohol abuse, head trauma, and so on. In such cases, the

Table 6.3. Sample cognitive screening batteries

I. Mini-Mental State Exam plus:
    Digit span
    Mesulam's cancellation tests
    Visual memory test
    Similarities
    Trailmaking tests
    Rey–Osterrieth figure or Hooper visual test

II. Mattis Dementia Rating scale plus:
    Months of the year backwards
    Clockface drawing
    Serial threes or simple arithmetic
    Map drawing

Note: Section II is for more impaired patients.

verbal subscore of the WAIS may remain unchanged while the performance score declines; the difference between the two scores increases with progression of the underlying problems. Normally, the two subscores should be within ten points of each other. For the elderly, age-corrected scaled scores can be used to compensate for the decline in performance ability associated with normal aging; if these age-corrected scales are used, verbal and performance IQ scores should remain equivalent. In some disorders, such as attention deficit disorder, the performance subscore on the WAIS may be much lower than the verbal sub-score. On the other hand, some conduct-disordered patients have lower verbal than performance scores; perhaps inadequate verbal skills make them more likely to "act out" their feelings in the form of behavioral problems rather than to think and talk through their feelings and frustrations. Dyslexics do worse on many verbal subtests than performance ones.

SCREENING TESTS

The *Mini-Mental State Exam* (Folstein, Folstein, and McHugh, 1975) is a brief, widely used screening test that superficially assesses several dimensions of language and cognitive functioning: orientation, registration, immediate recall, concentration, naming, articulation, construction, sentence writing, and three-stage command comprehension (see Table 6–4). It has a maximum score of 30 points, and unimpaired persons average 28 points. Scores of 24 or less are considered abnormal and indicate diffuse cognitive dysfunction. It is unfor-tunately not as sensitive as it is specific; that is, an abnormal score highly suggests that a problem is present, yet patients with milder forms of delirium or dementia may score 25 or more points, giving the false impression that they are cognitively intact. This is especially likely in highly intelligent persons with early dementia. Low scores in persons with less than eight years of education require cautious interpretation.

The *Mattis Dementia Rating Scale* (Coblentz et al., 1973; Mattis, 1976) is a screening test for patients who are expected to be incapable of performing more challenging tests—for example, demented or brain-injured patients. It has a total of 144 possible points, and scores below 124 are usually considered abnormal. Normative scores for the elderly are listed in Table 6–5. However, the total score is not as informative as are the five subscores: attention, construction, memory, initiation/perseveration, and conceptualization. Even though many clinicians use the Mattis in screening elderly patients at risk for dementia, it is deficient in screening for language problems. It is stronger in testing visuospatial abilities, memory, and attention. It tests for perseveration, and, unlike the Mini-Mental State Exam, it assesses conceptualization by using similarities and other abstrac-tion tasks. It is designed so that the most difficult task in any subsection is administered first; if the patient can perform the most complex task, then it is not necessary to continue to the easier tasks. It thus saves time.

Table 6.4. Mini-Mental State Examination

		Score	Points
Orientation			
1. What is the	Year?		1
	Season?		1
	Date?		1
	Day?		1
	Month?		1
2. Where are we?	State?		1
	County?		1
	Town or City?		1
	Hospital?		1
	Floor?		1
Registration			
3. Name three objects, taking one second to say each. Then ask the patient all three after you have said them. Give one point for each correct answer. Repeat the answers until patient learns all three.			3
Attention and Calculation			
4. Serial sevens. Give one point for each correct answer. Stop after five answers. Alternate: Spell **WORLD** backwards.			5
Recall			
5. Ask for names of three objects learned in Q.3. Give one point for each correct answer.			3
Language			
6. Point to a pencil and a watch. Have the patient name them as you point.			2
7. Have the patient repeat "No ifs, ands, or buts."			1
8. Have the patient follow a three-stage command: Take a paper in your right hand. Fold the paper in half. Put the paper on the floor.			3
9. Have the patient read and obey the following: **CLOSE YOUR EYES.** (Write it in large letters.)			1
10. Have the patient write a sentence of his or her own choice. (The sentence should contain a subject and an object and should make sense. Ignore spelling errors when scoring.)			1
11. Enlarge the design printed below to 1.5 cm per side, and have the patient copy it. (Give one point if all sides and angles are preserved and if the intersecting sides form a quadrangle.)			1

= TOTAL

_____
(30 maximum)

Source: Folstein, M. F., Folstein, S. E., and McHugh, P. R. Mini-Mental State: A Practical Method for Grading the Cognitive State of Patients for the Clinician. *Journal of Psychiatric Research* 12: 189–198, 1975. (Reproduced by permission from Pergamon Press Ltd.)

Table 6.5. Mattis dementia rating scale scoring system
for subjects ages 65–89 years

	Mean	SD
Total score	137.28	6.94
Attention	35.47	1.59
Initiation & perseveration	35.50	3.02
Construction	5.80	0.61
Conceptualization	37.25	2.58
Memory	23.28	2.12

Source: Spreen, O., and Strauss, E. *A Compendium of Neuropsycholog-ical Tests: Administration, Norms, and Commentary.* New York: Oxford University Press, 1991. (Reproduced by permission.)

ATTENTION AND CONCENTRATION TESTS

The *Trailmaking Tests Parts A and B* (Armitage, 1946; War Department, 1944; Reitan, 1958), are very useful for screening sustained attention (see Figure 6–8). In addition, they assess visuospatial and motor integrative function and cognitive flexibility (probably a prefrontal cortex function), both of which are required to switch quickly from numbers to letters. This is a timed test (in seconds), and

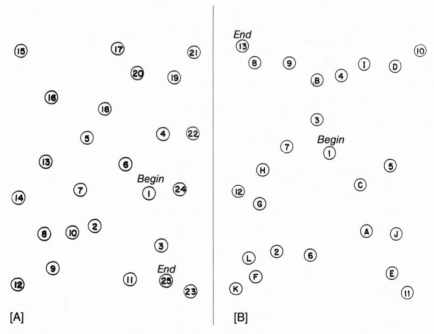

FIGURE 6–8 Trailmaking Tests Parts A and B, for assessing concentration, mental flexibility, and psychomotor speed. (War Department 1944; Armitage 1946; Reitan 1958)

there are different norms for various age groups (Lezak, 1983). For adults of age 70 years and under, it is reasonable to use 34 seconds as the upper limit for the normal range in Part A of the test, and 89 seconds for Part B during routine clinical use. In addition, Table 6–6 lists normative scores for different age groups. As with any timed test, the elderly usually perform more slowly. Part A consists of circled numbers that the patient must connect with lines in ascending order from number 1 to 25. Part B is similar, except that the patient must connect numbers and letters, alternating between them, in ascending order for numbers and the alphabet. Part B is especially sensitive in detecting diffuse cognitive dysfunction.

Mesulam's (verbal and nonverbal) cancellations tests (Mesulam, 1985; Figure 6–9A,B) involve timing the patient's performance and assessing accuracy in circling an intended item from among distractors. In the verbal form, the patient is instructed to circle all of the letter A's; and in the nonverbal form, to circle all of the open circles with the slanted line through them. There are 60 target symbols to circle on each form, with 15 per visual field (quadrant). Normal persons under 50 years of age should complete each form in under 2 minutes and without any errors; normals over 50 may be expected to miss up to one target per quadrant; and normals over 80 may be expected to miss up to four targets per quadrant (Mesulam, 1985). Patients with anosognosia will neglect the left side of the form, whereas those with visual field cuts will miss the affected quadrant(s).

Another test of concentration is the *Symbol Digit Modalities Test* (Smith, 1968). At the top of the form is a key, which is a row of symbols, each corresponding to a number from one to nine (see Figure 6–10). The remainder of the page consists of rows of symbols with empty boxes below each symbol in which the patient fills in the corresponding number, according to the key at the top of

Table 6.6. Trailmaking tests normative scores for different ages

Percentile	15–20 Years (n = 108)		20–39 Years (n = 275)		40–49 Years (n = 138)		50–59 Years (n = 130)		60–69 Years (n = 120)		70–79 Years (n = 90)	
	A	B	A	B	A	B	A	B	A	B	A	B
90	15	26	21	45	18	30	23	55	26	62	33	79
75	19	37	24	55	23	52	29	71	30	83	54	122
50	23	47	26	65	30	78	35	80	35	95	70	180
25	30	59	34	85	38	102	57	128	63	142	98	210
10	38	70	45	98	59	126	77	162	85	174	161	350

Note: Time in seconds (on parts A and B) for normal control subjects at different age levels.
Source: Spreen, O., and Strauss, E. A *Compendium of Neuropsychological Tests: Administration, Norms, and Commentary.* New York: Oxford University Press, 1991. (Adapted by permission.)

N X E A P W B V A Q H R Y A K O G M A Z L O
A F Z R U A T I L S C X E P W B A Q V D G A
Q I O G A V K Y D U A A B Z T F J A L R M C
B A L P K R A J E I O Z H V X A Q F W S A U
T J S A F M Z V A K L E U A R I H P A O B X
F N R E W C A H P Y Q M J S D A Z V K I G L
U A I Z X A O B L F T G P Y C W A E R H A N
L V A J P S R K I A B N A F X U M Q D A C W
O K Q D C M H W G E V R S B I L Z T Y F U J
Y Z A U T I G F S A J O A D P H N R M A E V
E A W H R A L T B M D V I G O S A K U X A P
R T P Y N K A S W L U C Q E H A F B J O Z I
H B K A G O C E A P R I W A U Q L D A T S Y
D A J S I L A N F R E P C H V A O G T B A K
C Q T B A E W O R J A A L I M D S A H G K F
A L G I D A S M K B F H R U E J A O P C N A
S E H A B W F P A G Z T K A Q Y R C A U I M

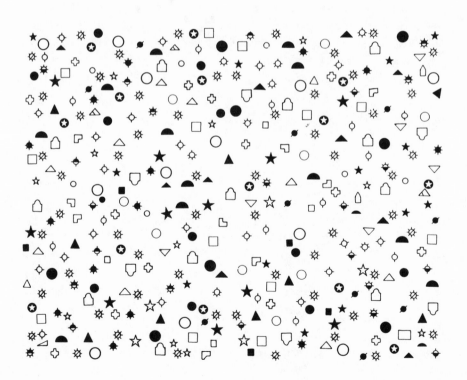

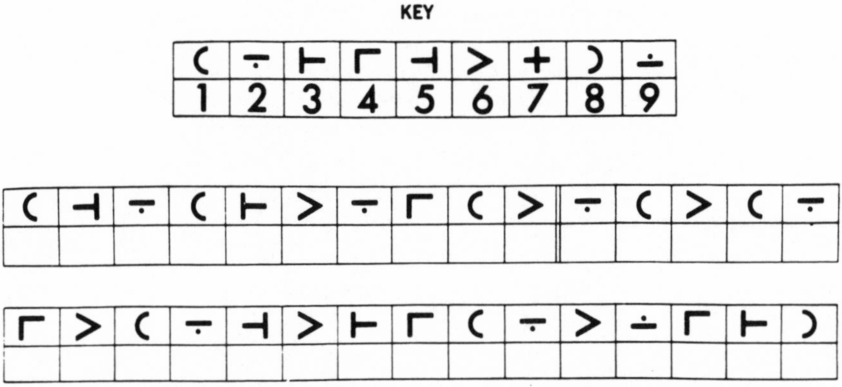

KEY

FIGURE 6–10   A section of the Symbol–Digit Modalities test for assessing concentration and cognitive flexibility. Copyright © 1973 by Western Psychological Services. Reprinted from the *Symbol Digit Modalities Test* by permission of the publisher, Western Psychological Services, 12031 Wilshire Boulevard, Los Angeles, California 90025.

the page. This is a timed test, with the score equaling the total number of correct answers in 90 seconds. Patients unable to write can instead say aloud the correct number for each symbol. Education and age affect the scores on this test; thus there are separate normative scores for different age groups (see Table 6–7).

A challenging test of selective attention and concentration is the *Stroop Color–Word Test* (Golden, 1968). It consists of three pages of 100 words each, arranged in columns of 20. On the first page are the words "red," "green," and "blue" printed in black ink in random order. The patient is asked to read aloud correctly as many words as possible in 45 seconds. The second page has X's arranged like the words on the first page, except each series of "x's" is printed in red, blue, or green ink. The patient reads aloud as many colors as possible in 45 seconds. The third page consists of similarly arranged words "red," "blue," or "green," each printed in ink of one of these three colors, but the ink color does not match the word (e.g., the word "red" is printed in *blue* ink). The patient is asked to read aloud the color of the ink for each word as quickly as possible in 45 seconds. For each page the score is the total number of correct responses. Obviously, the third page is the most difficult because word-reading is a highly overlearned ability that produces interference while one is trying to ignore the word and recite the colors.

←

FIGURE 6–9   Two of four subtests from Mesulam's cancellation tests, one for verbal and the other for nonverbal assessment of concentration. For Figure 6–9A *(top)*, the letter A is circled wherever it appears; for Figure 6–9B *(bottom)*, the symbol " ☼ " is circled. (Reproduced from Mesulam, M-M. *Principles of Behavioral Neurology*. Philadelphia: F. A. Davis, 1985, by permission of F. A. Davis, publishers.)

Table 6.7. Symbol digit modalities test normative scores (ages 18–74)

Age Group	Mean Education	Mean Written Administration	Mean Oral Administration
18–24 (n = 69)	12.7	55.2 (± 7.5)	62.7 (± 9.1)
25–34 (n = 72)	13.5	53.6 (± 6.6)	61.2 (± 7.8)
35–44 (n = 76)	12.1	51.1 (± 8.1)	59.7 (± 9.7)
45–54 (n = 75)	11.7	46.8 (± 8.4)	54.5 (± 9.1)
55–64 (n = 67)	11.3	41.5 (± 8.6)	48.4 (± 9.1)
65–74 (n = 61)	10.7	37.4 (± 11.4)	46.2 (± 12.8)

Source: (Based on studies by Carmen C. Centofanti) Spreen, O., and Strauss, E. A Compendium of Neuropsychological Tests: Administration, Norms, and Commentary. New York: Oxford University Press, 1991. (Reproduced by permission.)

Impulsive patients make many errors on this test. An alternative administration and scoring system for this test involves timing how long it takes to correctly read 100 items.

CONSTRUCTIONAL ABILITY AND VISUAL MEMORY

The *Rey–Osterrieth Complex Figure* drawing task (Osterrieth, 1944) is a particularly challenging test of constructional ability, which also evaluates organizational and perceptuomotor skills. Figure 6–11 shows this design. It has the basic shape of a rectangle that is further subdivided and then decorated with various lines. The patient is asked to copy it as accurately as possible onto a blank sheet of paper. A maximum of five minutes is allowed to complete the drawing. How the drawing is begun and executed is observed. Most normal persons quickly notice the rectangle and begin by drawing it, then subdivide it, and then add details, because beginning with the large rectangle helps to keep the design proportionate. Brain-damaged patients usually have a great deal of difficulty copying the drawing, and those with right hemisphere lesions usually miss the overall form (rectangle) and focus on smaller details, therefore drawing a disproportionate figure. Severely brain-damaged patients, especially those patients who have non-dominant hemisphere lesions, will draw something with little or no resemblance to the design. Figure 6–12 shows examples (A through E) from actual patients who have attempted to copy this design. The Rey–Osterrieth figure can also be used to test short-term visual memory. In this case, the patient is asked to redraw the design from memory after a brief delay; this recall task is sensitive to non-

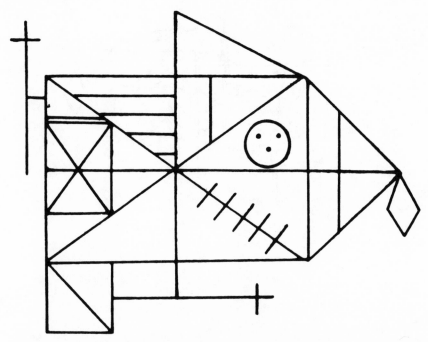

FIGURE 6–11 The Rey–Osterrieth Complex Figure for assessment of visuoconstructional ability as well as visual memory. (Reproduced from Osterrieth, P. A. Le test de copie d'une figure complexe. *Archives de Psychologie* 30: 206–356, 1944, by permission.)

dominant temporal-lobe dysfunction. To test long-term visual memory, the examiner tests for delayed recall after 30 minutes. There is a very specific scoring system for this test which can be found in the text by Spreen and Strauss (1991).

AGNOSIA, APRAXIA, AND ANOMIA

The *Mini Object Test* (Still, Goldschmidt, and Mallin, 1983) can be used to test for anomia, agnosia, and apraxia. It utilizes an inexpensive children's game called "Jack Straws," comprised of miniature plastic objects including a wrench, pitchfork, ladder, rifle, paddle, shovel, ax, and saw. The patient is asked to name each object and then to demonstrate how it should be used. The patient who does not visually recognize an object is allowed to feel it to identify it. *Anomics* are impaired in naming objects even though they can demonstrate their use; *agnosics* can neither recognize the objects nor describe their use; and *apraxics* can name and describe the use of the objects but cannot demonstrate their use. This test is scored on a 30-point scale and has been shown to differentiate demented from either depressed or schizophrenic patients. It can also be useful for the naming portion of language assessment (see Chapter 4).

A.

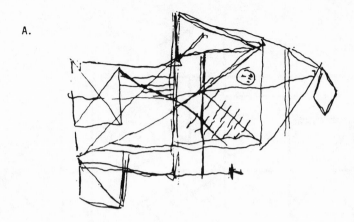

B.

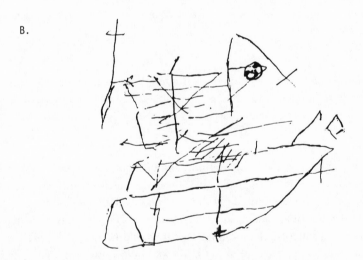

FIGURE 6–12   Several patients' attempts at copying the Rey–Osterrieth design. Patient A, previously an artist, had Alzheimer's dementia; the drawing was done piecemeal with many double lines (perseveration). Case B had bilateral, small parietal lobe strokes and parkinsonism; the drawing shows significant distortion and inaccuracies, as might be expected with parietal lobe lesions. Case C did not start with the rectangle and progressed

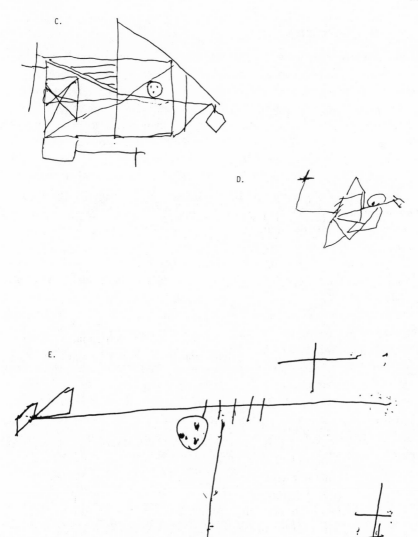

in a piecemeal fashion; the final product was basically correct, though it had some inaccuracies. Case D had dementia from hypothyroidism and pernicious anemia; the drawing is inadequate and small. This same patient drew the clockfaces A and D in Figure 6–6. Sample E is also very poor, drawn by a dementing patient who had complex visual hallucinations associated with Alzheimer's.

Integration of Findings

When cognitive deficits are found, the types of deficits should be listed and summarized in order to establish whether patterns exist that could give clues to etiology or differential diagnosis. For example, the patient might have deficits only in memory that would point toward an amnestic syndrome or early dementia. If the deficits are mostly attentional, and there seems to be a pattern of inconsistent performance even within a particular area, suggesting a motivational problem, then a depression-induced pseudodementia or mild/subclinical delirium might be considered. If many different areas are impaired, including orientation, attention, calculations, working memory, and long-term memory, then delirium or dementia should be considered. An older person's difficulty naming objects, memory deficits, and visuospatial problems in drawing or constructional tasks suggest early Alzheimer's dementia. Inattention on most tasks and short attention span suggest attention deficit disorder. Thus, the findings must be synthesized to determine their meaning and implications for clinical care.

When cognitive deficits are detected during the MSE, they may seem readily attributable to a particular syndrome, such as amnesia, dementia, stroke, delirium, or depression-induced pseudodementia. If not, it may be helpful to get an opinion from a psychologist, psychiatrist, or neurologist who is specially trained and qualified to administer and interpret neuropsychologic tests. Such tests are an extension of the simpler tests performed during the MSE. When and which patient to refer is a matter of clinical judgment, however.

Many standardized cognitive tests can be repeated at a later date, allowing objective comparison of findings. Because the patient may remember how to perform a particular test, equivalent and alternate forms of that test may need to be used for repeated testing (though not all tests are susceptible to practice effects). Learning how to perform a given type of test may account for improvement seen in scores over the first several times it is repeated. In addition, if a test is easy enough that a patient scores perfectly or nearly so, repeated testing may not be sensitive enough to detect improvement because of a *ceiling effect*, that is, the person cannot score any higher. It is best to choose tests that are challenging enough for a given patient so that improvement can be documented upon retesting.

Most MSE cognitive test findings need to be interpreted in light of the patient's level of education and intelligence. Elderly patients also need special consideration, as there is a normal decay in psychomotor speed with aging and because, as a cohort, they are less likely to have had the extended education that has become common in current generations. However, for example, a 70-year-old retired accountant can be expected to calculate better than most of his or her peers.

Definitions

Abstraction   The capacity for higher levels of thinking, which involves a conceptualization of ideas beyond the most obvious, concrete meaning of words. This includes the ability to make connections and comparisons between events or ideas that extend beyond the manifest content of words. This capacity involves synthesizing and analyzing information, as well as appreciating broader thematic or conceptual categories of information. Proverb interpretation and the description of similarities between things of the same category (e.g., shirts and coats are both clothes; apples and pears are both fruits) are ways to test abstraction. Damage to prefrontal cortices and/or their subcortical connections in the basal ganglia and thalamus commonly produces impairment in the ability to abstract.

Agnosia   The inability to recognize an object or a nonverbal symbol even though primary sensory pathways, such as vision and hearing, are intact. This is a perceptual problem rather than a verbal one. The patient cannot comprehend an object's function, even though it was previously familiar to him or her. The patient may hold and look at something inquisitively, not knowing what to do with it. Agnosia can be of different types (e.g., visual, tactile, and auditory, or for faces or colors). Agnosia should be differentiated from anomia. (See Confrontational naming, in this section, and under Naming in Chapter 4.) Finger agnosia, color agnosia, and visual-object agnosia are caused by lesions of the left hemisphere.

Amnesia   The inability to remember recently learned material or to recall material from the past, despite intact attentional abilities. This may be modality-specific (e.g., a relatively selective auditory or visual memory deficit) or confined to a particular time period. *Anterograde amnesia* refers to the period of time following the onset of memory difficulties (i.e., since the occurrence of the accident or an insult to the brain which caused impairment of new memory formation). *Retrograde amnesia* refers to inability to remember material from a period of time preceding the brain insult that caused the onset of the amnesia. Amnesia refers to a defect in memory or learning and, as a syndrome, does not refer to memory deficits that result secondarily from deficits in other cognitive processes such as language and visuoperceptual thinking. Recall of long-term memories is impaired in amnesia, whereas attentional, short-term, and procedural memory abilities are usually still intact. Anterograde amnesia usually predominates over retrograde. Language is intact, as is intelligence, except when the memory decline is secondary to dementia. Patients may confabulate when they cannot remember, particularly when amnesia is still relatively acute. The neural basis of memory function is not completely understood but probably involves temporal lobes, frontal lobes, and the limbic system, with ascending connections from the brainstem. Korsakoff's syndrome, usually related to alcohol abuse, is the most common example of an amnestic syndrome; these patients cannot learn or retain new information. Head trauma, Herpes encephalitis, anoxic encephalopathy, diencephalic damage following a ruptured anterior communicating artery aneurysm, and tumors of the third ventricle also cause amnestic syndrome. Dementias may initially present as isolated memory disorders. Concussions produce retrograde and anterograde amnesia, which may be only temporary. Amnesias due to a structural or physiologic insult to the brain must be differentiated from hysterical causes (e.g., conversion disorder and fugue states) and from psychologic repression of a memory.

Apraxia   The inability to perform volitionally previously learned purposeful movements even though strength, coordination, comprehension, and sensation are intact; yet these movements can be performed in situations when not willfully initiated. Apraxia is due to a poorly understood disorder of higher cortical function resulting in a partial or complete inability to execute certain motions volitionally. It can affect specific functions, like dressing or copying geometric designs (*constructional apraxia*). It may affect either simple or complex motions. The apraxic patient cannot demonstrate how to use objects in a purposeful way (e.g., combing with a hairbrush or buttoning a shirt). The person is aware of the difficulties. Apraxia can accompany dementias, strokes, and lesions affecting frontal, parietal, or temporal lobes.

Attention   The ability to focus aspects of one's consciousness on certain incoming sensory stimulation without undue distraction from competing stimuli. Attention is required before registration, learning, and remembering can occur. Paying attention is a necessary precondition for most other cognitive and intellectual functions. Thus, an attentional deficit might adversely affect performance on a variety of subtests of a given cognitive battery. Deficits in attention (*distractibility*) can be caused by many circumstances, including delirium, depression, fatigue, drug intoxications, attention deficit disorder, stroke, head trauma, anxiety, and dementias. The neuroanatomy of attentional mechanisms involves ascending brainstem pathways, cingulate gyrus, thalamus, frontal lobes, and parietal lobes.

Calculation ability   The ability to understand and utilize mathematical constructs and symbols, in contrast to verbal symbols and words. Calculating requires visual and cognitive recognition of symbols and figures, remembering tables of mathematical procedures, and sequencing the order of numbers. Mathematical ability can be tested by using addition, subtraction, or multiplication. Serial calculations performed "in one's head" are often used, not simply to assess mathematical abilities but also as a measure of concentration, as in testing serial seven subtractions from 100. *Acalculia* (dyscalculia) is the inability to solve mathematical problems. The localization of acalculia depends on the deficit involved: disturbed spatial ability, difficulty appreciating numbers as symbols, comprehension problems, and so on. Left cerebral hemisphere lesions cause dyscalculia related to loss of arithmetic sense or alexia, whereas right hemisphere lesions cause dyscalculia related to loss of spatial relations sense.

Cognition   The ability to use intellect, thought, and ideas to comprehend inner and outer realities. A combination of cortical functions is involved in cognition, which includes language, memory, attention, perception, judgment, reasoning, and recognition.

Concentration   The ability to sustain attention over a period of time, without becoming distracted or losing the train of thought. It is related to *vigilance*, which is the ability to pay attention in order to monitor events and stimuli over a period of time. Concentration can be impaired by organic brain dysfunction, depression, head injury, and any conditions that disrupt attentional ability. It can be affected by damage to the parietal and frontal lobes, cingulate gyrus, and ascending brainstem neuronal pathways.

Concrete thinking   The type of thought that is based on a literal conception of facts or tangible objects. There is an inability to think beyond the context of the current moment, or beyond the most overt meaning or experience to another (e.g., hypothetical) level of thought or time. There is no appreciation of subtler meanings, double-meanings, and so on. Proverbs and similarities are literally interpreted. Concrete thinking is a less developmentally advanced type of thought as compared to abstract thinking. Concrete thinking is normal in latency-age children (prior to puberty). It can be noted in patients with schizophrenia, mental retardation, delirium, dementia, and frontal lobe damage.

Confabulation   The fabrication of ideas and circumstances that are not consistent with reality; it usually accompanies severe memory dysfunction. Elaborate, fictitious stories about oneself or other people, places, and events can be confabulated, and yet the patient has no insight or ability to comprehend that the confabulated material is untrue, nor is he or she attempting to deceive others. Such a person is not aware of and cannot monitor his or her own verbal output for accuracy of content. There are two types of confabulation: spontaneous and provoked (Kopelman, 1987). Spontaneous confabulation, which is wide-ranging and grandiose and resembles delusions, occurs with severe lesions of the frontal lobes. Provoked confabulation, which is in response to questions about forgotten information, occurs with lesions of temporal and limbic areas. Confabulation should be differentiated from delusions (see Chapter 5), if possible. This may be virtually impossible when delusions are not focused or fixed to a particular idea, person, or circumstance, but are rather poorly formed and all-encompassing, as in delirium. Confabulation needs to be differentiated from fluent aphasia (see Chapter 4). Confabulation can occur with damage to brain areas such as the temporal lobes, frontal lobes, and limbic system/thalamus, or to the pathways that interconnect them. Tumor, stroke, aneurysm, and chronic alcohol abuse are common causes of confabulation.

Confrontational naming   The ability to, on demand, ascribe appropriate verbal labels to things or people whose function or familiarity are recognized. Confrontational naming refers to the procedure of showing an object (e.g., a comb or wristwatch) or a picture of an object to a patient and requesting that patient to name it or one of its parts. Confrontational naming is impaired (dysnomia or anomia) in Alzheimer's dementia and aphasia. The assessment of verbal memory is frequently problematic in the presence of significant anomia (see Chapter 4).

Constructional ability   The ability to draw, construct, or manipulate shapes and figures in two and three dimensions. It requires integration of occipital, parietal, and frontal lobe function. The left hemisphere contributes to the ability to draw details or specific things, whereas the right hemisphere perceives spatial configuration of the whole image.

Dementia   A global deterioration of cognitive and intellectual functions. Dementia is a diagnosis, not a single sign or symptom, and usually involves more symptoms than simply cognitive decline, such as changes in personality and mood, or the presence of psychotic symptoms. The diffuse cognitive dysfunction of dementia may begin in its earliest stages with a more focal type of cognitive deficit, but over time progresses to involve multiple functions. Depending on the type, different dementias can start with different symptoms, such as memory dysfunction, visuospatial deficits, personality change, or word-finding difficulty. There may be different patterns of deficits in "cortical" versus "subcortical" dementia, although both anatomic regions are probably affected to some degree in each category. Cortical pathology plays a major role in Alzheimer's, Pick's, and multiinfarct dementias, whereas clinical symptoms associated with subcortical pathology dominate the presentation in progressive supranuclear palsy, Huntington's disease, and parkinsonian dementias.

Declarative memory   Long-term memory for factual information about the world and one's own experience. It differs from procedural memory, which is related to perceptuomotor skills and "how to do" things. It includes verbal and nonverbal (pictorial) components. There are two types of declarative memory: semantic and episodic (see this section).

Episodic memory   The type of declarative, long-term memory that allows a person specifically to remember his or her own personal experiences from particular times in the past. It is related to semantic memory in that it builds on a base of general information, but differs from it in that it is a personalized knowledge of the world gained from that individual's own cumulative experiences. It is temporally related—that is, recalled in time—as in remembering attending a friend's birthday, remembering registering for the draft for the Vietnam War, and so forth. It is impaired in amnestic syndromes, some dementias, and often in head injury.

Graphesthesia   The ability, without looking, to perceive, recognize, and identify numbers or letters traced on the palm of the hand or on the palmar surface of the fingertips, through tactile stimulation. It is tested separately in each hand, usually using numbers from zero to nine. *Agraphesthesia*, or inability to identify such numbers, is a "soft" neurologic sign and, if unilaterally impaired, suggests dysfunction of the contralateral parietal lobe.

Long-term memory   Memory that is more permanent than short-term memory, covering a period of time ranging from days to years. Long-term memory may be affected even when short-term memory remains intact, suggesting that it is at least in part a separate neuroanatomic construct. Long-term memory can be categorized into *declarative* (informational or propositional) and *procedural* (motoric) memory, with declarative memory subdivided into *semantic* (general information) and *episodic* (time related) types (see Figure 6–2).

Orientation   The ability to understand and to be aware of one's self in relation to the environment, chronologic time or temporality, and one's own identity. Orientation is usually described for person, place and time. Disorientation usually occurs first for time, then for place, and then for person. Disorientation is common in delirium, severe amnesias, and moderately severe dementia; it may be seen in conversion and factitious disorders.

Perseveration   The persistent, inappropriate, and involuntary repetition of words, actions, or tasks. It often occurs even when circumstances or a request seem to require proceeding to a different task. This is usually beyond the patient's control and is seen in frontal lobe dysfunction, delirium, head trauma, schizophrenia, stroke, severe dementia, fluent aphasia, and other forms of brain damage (see Chapter 4).

Procedural memory   The type of long-term memory that relates to the acquisition of perceptual–motor skills—that is, learning how to perform certain specific skills such as driving a car or riding a bicycle. Amnestic patients are usually able to learn procedural skills, even though they would not be able to recall having done so and even though they have deficits in declarative memory.

Prospective memory   A type of long-term memory that allows a person to remember to do something at some particular future time. It is probably related to prefrontal cortex activity and is important in planning and organizing, as well as in staying oriented. It can also be affected in head injury and dementia, and is impaired early in delirium.

Pseudodementia   A pattern of cognitive deficits, especially involving memory, that mimics dementia from Alzheimer's or other known physical causes but that is associated with physiologically based disorders, such as major depression. It generally results from inattention, concentration deficits, and/or poor motivation to perform cognitive tasks. It may also be named for the condition with which it is associated (e.g., depression-induced dementia or dementia syndrome of depression). Pseudodementia can be seen in mania and in other psychiatric conditions (conversion disorder) as well. Because of attentional deficits and motivational impairments, it often produces diffuse cognitive deficits in an inconsistent and spotty pattern.

Registration   Functionally assessed as the ability to restate information immediately after it is presented. This ability is sensitive to attentional impairment. Registration of new information must occur before storage into memory or future retrieval can occur. The prefrontal cortex probably plays an important role in this ability.

Retrieval   The ability to recall information from memory; sometimes cues can be given to enhance retrieval. When cues are not given, it is called *free recall*. *Recognition* is a form of cued retrieval in which one is given multiple possible choices that include the target stimulus. When items can be associated into categories of similar items such as footwear, gems, modes of transportation, and so on, then learning and retrieval may be enhanced.

Semantic memory   A type of declarative, long-term memory that involves the acquisition of specific knowledge about the world at large, including history, vocabulary, and other factual knowledge learned at school or by reading, and so forth, as well as concepts and rules. An example is names of the U.S. presidents. Higher-level cognitive functioning is required to attain semantic memory, as opposed to procedural memory. In contrast to episodic memories, semantic memories are not time-tagged.

Short-term memory   A type of memory that is temporary and capacity-limited, and decays rapidly. It includes and requires the ability to pay attention, perceive, and recognize in order to register information. As such, it contrasts with long-term memory. Short-term memory involves the transient storage of information (registration) which then allows the person to learn, understand, and reason in a specific context. This short-term retention of information covers a time period of seconds or minutes. The term "short-term memory" is similar to, but not synonymous with, the terms "working memory" and "primary memory" which are used by researchers studying memory.

Soft neurologic signs A variety of motor or sensory impairments that are subtler than gross neurologic impairments and are indicative of central nervous system dysfunction, often of subcortical origin. They have low specificity for predicting neurologic disease and are often developmentally based. These signs include mirror movements, motor impersistence, agraphesthesia, astereognosis, and extinction to bilateral simultaneous stimulation. They may be useful in detecting dysfunction of frontal or parietal lobes in the absence of more robust deficits, and can be combined with detected cognitive deficits for possible localization of neuroanatomic lesions. This term is more often used by psychiatrists than by neurologists.

Stereognosis The ability to perceive, recognize, and identify objects placed in one's hand on the basis of tactile sensing of the shape of the object without seeing it. It is tested in each hand separately. Inability to perform this task is called *astereognosis*. This tests parietal lobe function.

Visuospatial ability The perceptual ability to comprehend visually the relationships of designs or structures in space, and to reproduce them. Adequate visual acuity is a prerequisite.

Word-finding difficulties The inability to recall words or names of things spontaneously during conversations or during confrontational naming. They occur in Alzheimer's dementia, in anxiety disorders, and with various other causes of inattentiveness, such as sleep deprivation. (See Confrontational naming in this section, and under Word-finding difficulty in Chapter 4).

References

Appelbaum, P. S., and Roth, L. H. Clinical issues in the assessment of competency. *American Journal of Psychiatry* 138: 1462–7, 1981.

Armitage, S. G. An analysis of certain psychological tests used for the evaluation of brain injury. *Psychological Monographs* 60: 1–48, 1946.

Army Individual Test Manual of Directions and Scoring. War Department, The Adjutant General's Office, 1944.

Coblentz, J. M., Mattis, S., Zingesser, L. H., Kasoff, S. S., et al. Presenile dementia. *Archives of Neurology* 29: 299–308, 1973.

Culver, C. M., and Gert, B. *Philosophy in Medicine: Conceptual and Ethical Issues in Medicine and Psychiatry.* New York: Oxford University Press, 1982.

Cutting, J. *The Right Cerebral Hemisphere and Psychiatric Disorders.* New York: Oxford University Press, 1990.

Folstein, M. F., Folstein, S. E., and McHugh, P. R. Mini-Mental State: A practical method for grading the cognitive state of patients for the clinician. *Journal of Psychiatric Research* 12: 189–98, 1975.

Fuster, J. M. *The Prefrontal Cortex: Anatomy, Physiology, and Neuropsychology of the Frontal Lobe* New York: Raven Press, 1980.

Golden, C. J. The Stroop Color and Word Test: A manual for clinical and experimental uses. Chicago: Stoelting, 1978.

Hecaen, H., and Albert, M. L. *Human Neuropsychology.* New York: John Wiley & Sons, 1978.

Hooper, H. E. *The Hooper Visual Organization Test: Manual.* Los Angeles: Western Psychological Services, 1958.

Kopelman, M. D. Amnesia: Organic and psychogenic. *British Journal of Psychiatry* 150: 428–42, 1987.

Lezak, M. D. *Neuropsychological Assessment,* 2nd edition. New York: Oxford University Press, 1983.

Mattis, S. Mental status examinations for organic mental syndrome in the elderly patient. In *Geriatric Psychiatry,* ed. L. Bellak and T. B. Karasu. New York: Grune & Stratton, 1976.

Mesulam, M.-M. *Principles of Behavioral Neurology.* Philadelphia: F. A. Davis, 1985.

Osterrieth, P. A. Le Test de copie d'une figure complexe. *Archives de Psychologie* 30: 206–356, 1944.

Reitan, R. M. Validity of the Trailmaking Test as an indicator of organic brain damage. *Perceptual Motor Skills* 8: 271–6, 1958.

Smith, A. The Symbol Digit Modalities Test: A neuropsychologic test for economic screening of learning and other cerebral disorders. *Learning Disorders* 3: 83–91, 1968.

Spreen, O., and Strauss, E. *A Compendium of Neuropsychological Tests: Administration, Norms, and Commentary.* New York: Oxford University Press, 1991.

Squire, L. R. Mechanisms of memory. *Science* 232: 1612–19, 1986.

Still, C. N., Goldschmidt, T. J., and Mallin, R. Mini Object Test: A new brief assessment for aphasia–apraxia–agnosia. *Southern Medical Journal* 76: 52–4, 1983.

Walsh, K. *Neuropsychology: A Clinical Approach,* 2nd edition. New York: Churchill Livingstone, 1987.

Williams, M. *Brain Damage, Behavior, and the Mind.* New York: John Wiley & Sons, 1979.

7 | Insight and Judgment

Insight and judgment are complex cognitive tasks that require the utilization and integration of several different mental functions, especially higher-level conceptual thinking. Prerequisites for insightfulness include the capacity for abstraction, ability to communicate (speech and language), intact cognitive function, absence of a thought disorder, euthymic mood, and stable affect (see Chapters 2 to 6). Even patients without disturbance of these functions may have poor insight as a result of using maladaptive psychologic defense mechanisms that distort the perception of internal and external realities or alter the motivation to relate openly with another person. In addition, the examiner needs to use his or her own abstract thinking in order to determine how insightful the patient is during the interview, because this determination is itself a subjective judgment. Evaluation of the patient's insight and ability to make sound judgments is based on both the content and the process of the interview (see Chapter 1). In general, the more severely ill a psychiatric patient is, the more likely it is that his or her capacity for insight will be impaired.

In order more fully to explore these constructs of insight and judgment, this chapter introduces the concepts of *defense mechanisms* and *personality*. These factors may adversely impact on decisionmaking and insight, even in the setting of intact language and cognition. Although there are slightly different psychoanalytic views about defense mechanisms and their definitions, we have chosen to mostly rely on Vallaint's (1977) descriptions. Even though specific personality styles or disorders are not documented in the MSE (but, rather, in the Assessment section of a written psychiatric evaluation because they represent diagnoses), predominant defense mechanisms should be described in the Insight and Judgment section of the MSE if they impact on the patient's capacity for attaining adequate insight and judgment about his or her illness and life events.

Insight and judgment are interrelated. The ability to make a sound judgment or decision presupposes an adequate level of insight. Insight requires taking a step back from oneself in order to evaluate critically the normalcy and repercussions of one's situation and behavior. Insight is the ability to be self aware—that is, conscious of one's own feelings, ideas, and underlying motivations about a particular issue (or about one's own psychologic condition). It involves the capacity to examine many aspects, viewpoints, and consequences of an issue before forming an opinion or making a decision. Insight includes thinking about the consequences of past or future decisions and actions, such as appreciating the effects on other persons, and, in this respect, requires some capacity for empathy.

Impulsive (as opposed to contemplative) decisionmaking is usually maladaptive and is generally not consistent with self-awareness. Impulsive behavior often has negative consequences. Inadequate insight and poor judgment are often evident in patients who act out their feelings, rather than verbalizing them and seeking mature resolutions. Sometimes adequately insightful persons still act impulsively if unconscious feelings interfere with a more appropriate course of action.

Insight is considered somewhat differently, depending on the therapeutic setting. For example, in psychoanalytic psychotherapy insight is a vital function and is therefore evaluated in detail; it requires the ability to look at oneself objectively, as an external observer would, and the desire to subject one's feelings and thoughts to scrutiny. However, for assessment purposes during the MSE, a more practical, expedient, and superficial notion is generally used. This involves an assessment of patients' capacity to acknowledge and appreciate their illness or problems and their comprehension of any associated implications or consequences. This notion of insight is as a cognitive or intellectual entity, in contrast to the insight that is emotionally perceived and gradually attained over time in the setting of psychodynamic psychotherapy. In psychodynamic psychotherapy the goal is a deep, multifaceted self-awareness. Psychotherapy involves serial uncovering of subconscious layers of conflictual thoughts, feelings, and defense mechanisms, that are painstakingly brought into conscious awareness with the help of a professionally trained psychotherapist.

A variable amount of insight precedes the formulation of an opinion or judgment. Judgment is a process that precedes formation of a decision or production of an action (see Figure 7–1). The psychiatrist can gather data about judgment by discussing past behaviors, decisions, and actions with the patient and comparing these "results" to the patient's understanding of the judgment that preceded them. Judgment is affected by an individual's level of insight, cognitive abilities, intelligence, thinking processes, mood, personality, and life circumstances. Perhaps even more than insight, judgment is affected by cultural and societal factors. The determination of the appropriateness of a patient's judgments is subjective, and is evaluated both in the context of societal standards and norms and also in comparison to the examiner's own judgments.

For simple decisions, the determination of the appropriateness of patients' judgments is straightforward. For example, most people would agree that it is a sound judgment to avoid crossing the street while the oncoming traffic has a green light. For more complex decisions, the attribution of the soundedness or rationality of the judgment preceding them becomes less simple. For example, a terminal cancer patient with widespread metastases may refuse chemotherapy, a decision based on a judgment that might be viewed as rational even in a society that usually precludes suicide.

The MSE interview permits assessment of the patient's judgments regarding

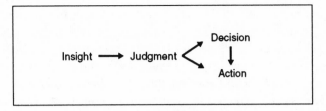

FIGURE 7–1   Relationship among insight, judgment, decision and action.

his or her condition and need for treatment, as well as the quality of the patient's everyday life decisions. Though the examiner cannot predict an individual's future judgments or actions (some would like to have us believe otherwise, particularly in the cases of future violent behavior), it is relevant to try to recognize an individual's usual patterns of formulating judgments. With this information, the treating psychiatrist may be able to help the patient gain insight into how and why such judgments are formed, thereby building a framework for possibly improving future judgments, decisions, and behaviors.

Whether individuals have good insight and judgment does not usually determine whether they are held responsible for their actions and decisions. Patients are responsible for their own actions except under rare circumstances (e.g., severe psychosis).

Application

Insight

Insight is the ability to be aware of internal (one's mind) and external realities (the environment, other people) to the extent that they are knowable. This implies that even subtle nuances, meanings, symbolisms, feelings, and thoughts are available to conscious awareness. Insight begins with awareness of and understanding of one's own feelings, thoughts, and reactions to other people or situations. After this self-reflection, insight requires comparison of how one feels and thinks about an issue or problem with what other people feel and think; this permits conscious awareness of one's conformity or nonconformity with societal norms. Thus, insight is the awareness of how one's own personality traits and behaviors contribute to symptoms, interpersonal problems, and so on. A psychologically mature person should have the capacity to be insightful.

From a practical perspective during the MSE, assessment of insight focuses on whether patients recognize that they are ill, comprehend that their problems are deviations from normal, understand that their behavior may affect others, and appreciate that treatment may be helpful in alleviating symptoms. This information is elicited through direct questions, for example: "Are you ill?" "What has brought you to see me?" "Have you had thoughts that other people view as abnormal, or are not normal for you?" "Do you realize that your family thinks you have been depressed?" "If you leave the emergency room without treatment for this chest pain, what will happen to you?" "What do you think is wrong with you?" "Do you think there is anything that will help you feel better?"

However, insight is a complex construct and not a single, easily quantifiable or anatomically localizable function of the human mind. Adequate insight presupposes intact intellectual and cognitive function, yet it is not synonymous with IQ. A highly intelligent person does not necessarily have good insight. Insight has emotional components, is somewhat culturally bound, and is impacted upon by one's defense mechanisms and personality style. Certain unconscious feelings may impede self-awareness. There are many aspects of self-awareness, including one's own psychologic state, social circumstances, medical condition, and so forth; an individual's degree of insight may be better for some of these areas than for others.

Adequate insight is usually vital for compliance with ongoing treatment and for informed consent. Insight itself may fluctuate with stress (e.g., the usually insightful but frightened patients with an acute myocardial infarction may deny the seriousness of her chest pain and try to leave the emergency room against medical advice) or with the current severity of psychiatric illness (e.g., the patient who does not realize, when manic, that his hypersexual behavior at church is inappropriate, but later when euthymic is embarrassed and remorseful). A persons' predominant defense mechanisms may also vary with the circumstances, thereby affecting his or her capacity for insight. For example, during an episode of mania, a person may use defense mechanisms of projection and denial, yet use more mature defense mechanisms when euthymic.

Informed consent in the medical setting often requires a patient to make a judgment and a decision about a proposed procedure; and that, in turn, requires a certain level of knowledge and insight regarding the nature of the procedure, risks and benefits, side or adverse effects, possible complications, and consequences of foregoing the procedure. Anything that prevents the insight component may impede the establishment of a completely "informed" consent. Common obstacles to achieving adequate insight include cognitive deficits, depressed or manic mood, and psychosis (see Table 7–1). As examples, a patient with Alzheimer's dementia may be unable to give informed consent for a necessary prostate resection because memory deficits prevent his learning about risks and benefits; a depressed patient may devalue her life, thus impeding realistic consideration of the risks and benefits of ECT treatment; a schizophrenic man who is delusionally persuaded that he is female seeks a sex change operation to which he cannot competently consent. Exhaustive technical knowledge on the part of the patient is not necessarily required for informed consent; thresholds vary according to the gravity and risks associated with the decision (see Chapter 6).

Table 7.1. Examples of disorders
whose symptoms may contribute to impaired
insight and judgment

Drug and alcohol dependence
Depression
Mania
Psychosis
Anxiety disorders
Personality disorders
Dementia
Delirium
Attention deficit disorder
Impulse control disorders
Obsessive-compulsive disorder
Central nervous system disorders
Conversion disorder
Factitious disorder

Persons who use psychotic, immature, and neurotic defense mechanisms are less capable of achieving full insight than are those who utilize mature mechanisms. Actively psychotic patients with paranoid schizophrenia often do not appreciate that they are mentally ill or how treatment can be helpful. Manic patients are usually so immersed in their elated or hyperactive state that they are not aware of or do not care about how their behavior affects others; they may be having so much fun that they do not realize they are behaving abnormally relative to their usual selves or to society. Manics and narcissistic personality-disordered persons tend to be grandiose about their capabilities, thereby diminishing their ability to be realistically aware of their condition or their limitations.

Extreme lack of insight is associated with conversion disorder (a dissociative state), factitious disorder, addictive disorders, and psychoses. By its very nature, conversion disorder implies a lack of conscious awareness of the underlying psychologic conflict that is masked and/or symbolized by the presenting somatic symptom. In factitious disorder, patients purposefully portray illness, yet are not conscious of their own motivations for being a patient. Psychosis from any cause involves psychotic and immature defense mechanisms that are not compatible with being insightful—for example, projecting onto another person one's own feelings (believing that the doctor has sexual feelings for the patient, when the converse is true), denial of reality in the face of otherwise notable data (a patient who believes she is dead), or delusional ideation (a patient who believed he called the football plays via television for a Steelers game).

Alcoholics and drug abusers frequently deny their addictions and the consequences thereof, externalize blame, do not take responsibility for themselves, and vigorously resist others' efforts to confront the problem. *Externalization* involves the use of external factors to rationalize actions instead of acknowledging internal impulses or feelings, for example: "I stayed at the bar all night because my old lady would have been on my case the second I came home"; rather than "I stayed at the bar all night because I can't control my urge to drink."

Many personality-disordered persons have inadequate insight into their disturbed relationships, thinking, and feelings, and are often resistant to changing these patterns. Borderline personality-disordered patients often use "black and white thinking" in which people or events are viewed as extremely good or bad, without awareness of "gray" zones of relativeness. This type of thinking is obviously not conducive to gaining full awareness of an issue or situation with appreciation of nuance, details, and ambiguity, and tends to lead to *splitting* (see Chapter 2, under Attitude) people into either good or bad. Severely depressed, suicidal patients have negatively distorted views of the world and themselves, which then diminishes their ability to appreciate the positive aspects of living.

Demented, delirious, amnestic, and brain-injured patients (e.g., stroke, head trauma) are all cognitively impaired; because of their attentional, memory, language, or abstraction deficits, these patients are often not capable of being insightful. Frontal lobe damage from alcohol, stroke, surgery, or head trauma directly alters executive functions (see Chapter 6, under Abstraction and Conceptualization), thereby reducing the capacity for conceptual thinking and self-knowledge. Thus, virtually any psychiatric disorder has the potential for impairing insight to some degree, though for a wide variety of reasons, including effects on cognition, mood, thought processes, language, and personality. Even a highly intelligent person may have poor insight secondary to psychiatric symptoms.

Insight should be viewed along a continuum, with many degrees between the extremes of insightfulness and lack of insight. *Anosognosia* is an example of extreme lack of insight, often the result of nondominant parietal lobe damage. Anosognosic patients typically deny suffering the functional impairment from their brain damage; when the paralyzed left arm is held in front of them, they may not recognize it as their own arm. Those who have significant prefrontal lobe damage from stroke, tumor, subcortical lesions, or head trauma also often lack insight and may even be disinhibited.

An otherwise insightful person might have a "blind spot" for a particular aspect of an issue or a specific topic. Intense religious beliefs may prevent flexible thinking and complete appreciation of an issue, especially in fundamentalistic religions that utilize strict, concrete interpretations of liturgy or teachings that are not conducive to alternate or abstract modes of thinking. Another example of a patient with incomplete insight is that of a mildly depressed attorney who describes a repetitive pattern of dating self-centered men, but cannot comprehend why she has not yet had an emotionally intimate relationship leading to marriage. She blames herself for being defective. Her mother is narcissistically impaired, and the patient has unconsciously spent her adult life seeking to conquer and secure affection from narcissistic men as she was never able to from her mother, but cannot herself recognize this connection. Another type of incomplete insight is minimization of illness—for example, the cavalier adolescent diabetic patient who intermittently doesn't comply with insulin requirements and dietary restrictions, or the recurrently depressed person who decides to stop taking antidepressant medication because he or she feels fine. At an intellectual level, such patients understand the increased risk for relapse, but may rationalize their situation with a variety of excuses. A multiple sclerosis or conversion-disordered patient may exhibit *la belle indifférence* (see Chapter 3, under Mood) which, by definition, impairs insight into the illness. In dementia, cognitive deficits generally impair insightfulness.

The most basic evaluation of patients' insight into their illnesses involves assessing the ability to agree that they are ill, that they may need further evaluation or testing, that they may benefit from treatment (including medication), and that they may have a higher risk for deterioration or relapse if they don't comply with treatment. While assessing these "here and now" illness-related issues, the examiner may also develop an understanding of the patient's prior capacity for insight from information not directly related to their illnesses. Questions about their approach to major life stresses, including relationships, past illnesses, family conflicts, and occupational issues, can help to elucidate the level of self-awareness. Sample questions are: "How did you cope with your wife's death?" "What did you do to keep from punching your boss?" "How do you handle your children when they skip school?" "How long did it take you to get to the emergency room after your chest pain began?" "When you had that headache as a medication side effect, did you call your doctor or stop taking the drug on your own?" and "Did you stop drinking when you were diagnosed with liver disease?" Such questions may elicit information about typical approaches and defensive styles in coping with life's problems and may offer a sneak preview of how a patient may view or cope with a current psychiatric illness. Patients' ability to take responsibility for optimizing their mental and physical health and compliance with treatment recommendations is significantly affected by their capacity for insight.

Because there are varying levels and types of insight, a thorough mental status report should document details about the examiner's assessment of the patient's insight, depending on the clinical situation. "Insight is nil" is not substantiated; better is "Insight is impaired, the patient denies any symptoms and blames the hospitalization on her parents." Other examples are: "The patient has relatively good insight into her illness and need for treatment, stating that her constant handwashing is injuring her skin and irritating her husband"; "Insight is limited; he recognizes that he is unhappy but feels his frequent angry outbursts are justified and the victims 'got what they deserved'"; "The patient appears to have deep psychological insight, describing how she learned from her parents to deal with men by flirtation and to dodge unwanted demands by verbally agreeing and then failing to follow through."

Judgment

Judgment is a process of consideration and formulation regarding a particular issue or situation that can lead to a decision or action. The better and more complete the person's insight, the more likely the judgment is to be sound, especially in complicated matters. Because insight and judgment are related to each other, much of the above discussion on insight applies to judgment as well. Although a snap judgment may happen to be a sound one, usually more contemplation is needed to produce a good judgment.

Judgment involves weighing and comparing the relative values of different aspects of an issue. Sound decisions are usually predicated on having made a comparison of pros and cons, and then concluding the way a "rational person" would in such circumstances. A judge on the bench engenders an image of a mature, thoughtful, calm presence in the courtroom, one who can be trusted to carefully consider various sides of a story and keep in mind what the laws and precedents of that society have recommended in the past. We trust that such a judge makes sound determinations. Similarly, everyone makes judgments in everyday life, either impulsively or based on some degree of contemplation, and the soundness of these judgments can be evaluated. Because judgments vary in their degree of complexity, the extent of weighing and consideration required also varies. Even in emergent situations requiring quick judgments, the capacity to integrate relevant information and take rapid action involves the same components as in more contemplative judgments—just more rapidly.

The ability to make sound judgments requires adequate insightfulness, intact cognitive function, capacity to conceptualize, sensitivity to the impact and consequences of a decision, ability to consider long-term effects and possible adverse outcomes, and appreciation of what a "rational" person in society would do. Any impairment of these functions diminishes the quality of the resultant judgment. People who tend to *act out* their feelings or ideas are prone to make judgments that are poorly thought out; often these people have difficulty conceptualizing and thinking deeply because their verbal skills are inferior to their performance skills; this occurs in the attention deficit-disordered child or adult, for example. People who behave impulsively and with minimal forethought are also likely to produce hasty judgments with resultant negative consequences; those who have personality disorders fall into this category.

Determining whether a particular judgment is sound is situation dependent. While killing other persons is considered immoral and a bad decision in most societies, an exception is made for a soldier in battle. Suicide attempts are usually considered abnormal and evidence of poor judgment in our society, but are more acceptable in some other societies and less aberrant in our society when persons are in severe pain from terminal illness.

Judgment is a process that precedes the outcome (decision or action). Even if the process of judgment is sound, the outcome can be bad. A person with sound judgment may have a poor outcome if poor frustration tolerance or an inability to delay gratification results in a premature or impulsive decision or action. Coercion by others may alter the resultant decision of an otherwise sound judgment. Conversely, good decisions or actions can occasionally occur even in the absence of a preceding, well-formed judgment if the person behaves in a knee-jerk fashion or, by chance, does the "right" thing. For example, an actively psychotic schizophrenic patient goes to the psychiatric emergency room seeking a cigarette and a cup of coffee; hospitalization results in order to treat the psychosis. In this case, the patient had poor insight and judgment, but happened to take correct action by going to the emergency room.

Judgment may be impaired as a consequence of impaired insight from the neuropsychiatric effects of intoxication with drugs or alcohol, as evidenced by the many persons who confidently drive their cars while intoxicated (see Table 7–1). It is likely that alcohol-dependent persons have impaired judgment even in the nonintoxicated state such that they complicate their lives by drinking in the first place. Judgment is impaired in depressed patients when negative and pessimistic feelings distort reality; this may even culminate in suicidal acts. Manics are insensitive to others' feelings and have poor judgment regarding their social behaviors; they often insult or embarrass others by their jokes or actions. Manics who are euphoric have an unrealistically happy view of the world and do not recognize potential negative consequences of their behaviors. Therefore, they may go on spending sprees when they have insufficient funds to pay for the purchases; engage in socially improper behaviors such as parading nude on their front lawns; or self-assuredly risk harm to themselves, such as when driving too fast or provoking fights they cannot win.

Patients with attention deficit disorders cannot maintain their attention long enough to focus their thinking and may behave impulsively. In contrast, obsessive patients spend a great deal of time thinking, yet have difficulty formulating judgments because they get caught up in details or are rigidly bound by rules. After brooding and ruminating for days, obsessive persons may force themselves to make a decision, only to finally make the "wrong" one. Schizophrenics who are actively psychotic may not be fully capable of sophisticated decision making because of delusions, thought disorder, or unrealistic distortions due to referential thinking.

Certainly, a delirious or demented patient who has significant cognitive deficits cannot be expected to make a sound, informed decision. Patients who have prefrontal cortex damage have difficulty with higher-level conceptualization, impeding their capacity to reason at an abstract level, or they may be disinhibited and impulsive. (*Disinhibition* is the loss of self-restraint or internal monitoring of behavior, resulting in socially inappropriate behaviors, such as publicly masturbating or telling profane jokes in genteel company.) Huntington's disease patients are often disinhibited and have difficulty with higher-level conceptualization, as in a frontal lobe syndrome. Mentally retarded persons are usually not capable of abstract thinking, thereby limiting their capacity to form judgments; they often also lack adequate appreciation for the nuances of social interactions and expectations. Stroke patients may have damage to areas of the brain required for language, cognition, or executive functions and thereby be less capable of making sound judgments.

It should be evident from the above discussion that a host of psychiatric and neurologic disturbances can reduce the capacity for making judgments; however, it must also be recognized that there are many potential degrees of reduction in the capacity to formulate judgments. The degree of importance of a required decision or action will vary, allowing for a range of what is considered a sound judgment depending on what is at stake. Most patients, even those who are unable to execute complex planning and choosing, are usually capable of understanding more basic and essential aspects of "right and wrong" or "good and bad," such as societal proscriptions against stealing or murdering. For example, although it is safe to assume that most murderers have a disturbance of judgment at some level, there are few "not guilty by reason of insanity" verdicts, at least in part because even moderately psychiatrically impaired persons are judged capable of making basic judgments, such as the wrongness of murder.

There are cultural, societal, religious, and ethnic differences regarding what is considered to be a rational or acceptable judgment. Simultaneously seeking help from a root doctor and a traditional physician makes sense to patients who believe in both types of healing. A desperate cancer victim who travels to Mexico to obtain Laetrile could be viewed as not making a good decision by those unaffected by cancer. On the basis of religious beliefs, some patients refuse blood transfusions during surgery despite the increased risk for mortality. Such a decision would be viewed as ludicrous by those members of society who do not share the religious objection to accepting transfusions.

Traditionally, students learning the MSE have been taught to ask certain questions to assess a patient's judgment. These include: "If you found a stamped, addressed letter on the street, what would you do with it?" or "If you were in a crowded movie theater and you were the first one to notice a fire, what would you do?" The expected appropriate answers would be "I'd put it into a mailbox" and "I would calmly go for help," respectively. Incorrect responses include "I'd throw it away" or "I'd open it to see what's inside" for the letter question, and "I would stand up and scream 'Fire!'" or "I'd run out yelling 'Help, fire!'" for the theater question. These simple and easily understood hypothetical situations provide a rudimentary assessment of judgment but are often inadequate to assess patients' judgments regarding complex situations that are faced in everyday life.

A more illuminating approach is to question patients about current difficulties, the issues they are contemplating in regard to an upcoming decision, or the way in which they handled past situations. This must be individualized, and therefore, the use of a stock question is not possible; nevertheless, judgment can usually be directly or indirectly assessed during interview questioning. Questions like "What do you think we should do about these hallucinations you are having?" or "How will you explain to your spouse your decision to sell drugs to pay for the new car?" or "Could you try to imagine and describe to me who would attend your funeral if you killed yourself, and how they would react?" or "What makes you think that you won't take this medicine that I have prescribed for you?" or "If you had a magic wand and could wave it to change your situation in any way you wanted, what would your life be like?"

Patients' judgments and decisions about complying with treatment may be similar to how they approach other decisionmaking. A patient might say, "I know I should take that medicine for my asthma so that I can breathe easier, but I just don't like taking pills for any medical problem." A person's defensive style can greatly affect his or her judgments; the more mature styles increase the likelihood of making rational judgments. Denial, projection, repression, externalization, and dissociation adversely affect judgment, whereas humor, altruism, and suppression are less likely to interfere. At the very least, it is important to establish to what extent patients think they can comply with the recommended treatments and interventions that the health care providers believe are in their best interest.

Defense Mechanisms

Defense mechanisms are psychologic maneuvers that attempt to mitigate unpleasant or undesired thoughts and feelings, or to cope with external forces. Individuals may employ more than one defense mechanism, and one's repertoire may change with time. There are a number of such mechanisms (see Table 7–2), many of which are described in detail in the Definitions section of this chapter. They vary in their level of maturity and adaptiveness. Mature defense mechanisms include *altruism, humor, sublimation,* and *suppression. Repression, displacement, dissociation, reaction formation* and *intellectualization* are examples of neurotic defenses. *Splitting, externalization, idealization, projection,* and *acting out* are immature defenses, whereas *denial* and *distortion* are psychotic defenses. The more mature the level of defense mechanisms utilized by a particular patient, the more likely that that person has the capacity for adequate insight and formulation of sound judgments. By the same token, the more immature or psychotic the defense mechanisms utilized, the less likely that that person will be capable of being insightful and making sound judgments. An

Table 7.2. Hierarchy of defense mechanisms

Mature types
Altruism
Humor
Sublimation
Suppression
Neurotic types
Repression
Displacement
Dissociation
Reaction formation
Intellectualization
Immature types
Splitting
Externalization
Idealization
Projection
Acting out
Psychotic types
Denial
Distortion

Source: Adapted from Vaillant, G. E. *Adaptation to Life: How the Best and the Brightest Come of Age.* Boston: Little, Brown, 1977.

actively psychotic patient who has persecutory delusions may be cognitively intact but may not be able to appreciate the need for an invasive medical procedure because of projection, distortion, and denial. A borderline personality-disordered patient may project onto others his or her own shortcomings, thereby precluding healthy relationships. An alcoholic patient may externalize blame for financial losses onto a spouse, denying the impact of the addiction and thereby rejecting the need to attend a rehabilitation program.

For the purpose of the MSE, specific mention of defense mechanisms is generally not required, unless they are particularly relevant to the patient's current situation or condition. For example, mention of defense mechanisms should be made when there is a striking repetitious pattern, when they impede the patient's cooperation with the MSE, when they impact significantly on the current crisis or complaint, and before embarking on psychoanalytic psychotherapy. For a borderline personality-disordered patient, an example would be "manipulates, projects, and splits"; for an obsessive-compulsive patient, would be "intellectualizes and displaces." When defenses are mentioned, they should be recorded and integrated into the Insight and Judgment section of the MSE report.

Definitions

Acting out   An immature and maladaptive defense mechanism in which the person expresses an unconscious impulse through a motor act, instead of becoming consciously aware of the emotion and then verbalizing it. Chronic self-abuse, such as superficially cutting oneself, is an example of acting out one's feelings of helplessness, anger, need for attention, self-hate, and so on. It is an indirect, and often manipulative, way to express one's needs or desires. An adolescent who craves parental attention may crash the family car or repeatedly come home after curfew, in order indirectly (but not adaptively) to have his or her needs met. Conduct-disordered children and borderline and antisocial personality-disordered adults often act out their feelings, usually with negative consequences—for example, rebellious and illegal activities, or suicidal gestures.

Altruism   A mature defense mechanism in which the person gains gratification and satisfaction from helping others. This does not include *masochism*, a more primitive process in which the person sacrifices him- or herself and receives pain or hardship in return. In *altruism*, the reward for good deeds may be feeling better about oneself. It is adaptive because both the giving and receiving parties realize a direct and concrete benefit. Persons with healthy, mature personalities utilize altruism as a defense mechanism.

Anosognosia   A neurologic term for the denial of illness, including the inability to recognize part of one's body, or its impairment, or a nearby physical space. The patient may neglect or deny the existence of the affected body part or an object in the affected area. It is usually seen accompanying right hemisphere lesions affecting the parietal lobe. Patients with such lesions ignore the left half of their bodies or visual fields. Bilateral frontal lobe lesions can also produce anosognosia, as can bilateral occipital lobe lesions (Anton's syndrome) and many amnesias. Anosognosia is an example of extreme inattention or lack of awareness (insight).

Defense mechanisms   Psychologic mechanisms of adaptation to stress and the environment. The psyche needs to be protected from adverse factors, much like the body is protected by wearing clothing or armor. Defense mechanisms are attempts to protect against both internal and external adversity. They help to control impulses that may have adverse consequences for the individual, and to minimize or avoid the emotionally painful or conflictual effects of reality, including in interpersonal relationships. Painful emotions include feelings of guilt, sadness, loss, anxiety, danger, shame, and rejection. There is a maturation process consisting of stages of personality development during which the "healthy" individual uses predominantly certain types of defense mechanisms (see Table 7–2). According to Vallaint (1977), this maturation process progresses from using *psychotic defenses* (normal in preschool children and in dreams, but abnormal in adults, such as when they occur in psychotic persons) to using *immature defenses* (normal in children and young adolescents, but abnormal in adults, such as when they occur in personality disorders), to using *neurotic defenses* (common in adults, especially during stress), to using *mature defense mechanisms* (common in psychologically healthy adults). It is expected in normal development that as a person psychosocially matures, he or she will gradually utilize more mature defense mechanisms in coping with everyday life. During times of great stress, however, people may temporarily revert back to using less mature defense mechanisms (known as *regression*, such as to more dependence during a medical illness). Immature defense mechanisms are employed by personality-disordered persons. Psychotic defense mechanisms are utilized by persons who have primary process thinking and thought disorder (see Chapter 5), including schizophrenics, manics, psychotic depressives, and severe personality-disordered patients, especially borderlines.

Denial A psychotic defense mechanism in which the person refuses to acknowledge the external reality of something, even in the face of convincing evidence. This denial of the existence of something, or of some experience may be of delusional proportions. (See anosognosia, under Constructional Ability in Chapter 6; and Delusions, in Chapter 5.) While somewhat related to repression (see below, this section), denial is much more intense and abnormal, and it persists even though it contradicts external reality as perceived by normal persons. This is a primitive thinking process, and may occur in severe personality disorders and psychoses, and occasionally in normal persons under great stress— for example, in a patient with an acute myocardial infarction who insists on leaving the emergency room and cannot be convinced that he had a heart attack; or, a schizophrenic patient who accuses others of stealing her underwear, but when the hospital staff observes her putting it under her mattress, she denies that it is hers.

Displacement A neurotic defense mechanism in which the person redirects his or her feelings toward a less important person or thing. For example, after a bad day at work, the displacer arrives home and kicks the dog, instead of having been assertive with his or her boss. Practical jokes and wit, which can be biting, may express displaced emotions.

Dissociation A neurotic defense mechanism in which the personality is temporarily altered to avoid emotional distress. Conversion disorders and fugue states are examples of escaping (dissociating) from one's usual self-awareness because of an upsetting event or feeling. Dissociation is not a healthy response to adversity because the precipitating psychologic conflict is not available for conscious awareness, understanding, or resolution.

Externalization A tendency to blame events, persons, or organizations external to oneself for the things that occur in or affect one's life. Inherent in externalization is the inability to take responsibility for one's own feelings, actions, decisions, and behaviors. An immature defense mechanism related to projection and denial, externalization is the predominant defense mechanism used by alcoholics and other drug-dependent persons, as well as by some personality-disordered persons.

Humor A mature defense mechanism in which playful or funny ideas are used to diffuse tense or unpleasant feelings, but not at the expense of another person's feelings. Humor makes it easier consciously to address conflictual or painful emotions or topics.

Insight The ability to be aware of subtle meanings of thoughts, ideas, and feelings, particularly as they relate to oneself. Insight is generally associated with more mature levels of personality development and defense mechanisms (e.g., sublimation, humor, altruism, and suppression) and is dependent on having both intact cognitive and intellectual functions, particularly of the prefrontal lobes (see Chapter 6), and the capacity for secondary process thinking (see Chapter 5). An insightful person can utilize knowledge, integrate it, and interpret it, using higher-level conceptual thinking. In its most practical definition, as used for the MSE, insight is the ability to acknowledge the presence of psychiatric symptoms and the possible need for treatment. A different definition of insight is the ability to be aware of deeply held previously unconscious feelings, usually recognized with guidance during psychotherapy.

Intellectualization A neurotic defense mechanism in which the person thinks about and analyzes ideas while remaining emotionally distant from or not recognizing accompanying feelings. On the surface, it appears that the patient has a clear and detailed understanding of an issue but does not experience or recognize the emotional components. The intellectualizing person will sound bland and analytic when relaying what should be an affect-laden topic. This defense mechanism is commonly used by persons with obsessive-compulsive personality styles.

Judgment The process of forming an opinion or conclusion based on information about a situation and, ideally, reaching a conclusion that appropriately weighs and recognizes the important elements of an issue. Judgment is a subjective phenomenon. Judgment is affected by intellect, the quantity or quality of data available concerning a particular decision to be made, personality, past experience, mood, feelings, cognitive abilities, cultural/subcultural and societal factors, and any extrinsic factors bearing on the possible decision outcomes (e.g., coercion). Judgment is also affected by insight and the ability to use abstract thinking. Intact frontal lobe function, especially of the prefrontal cortex (see Chapter 6), is necessary for higher-level judgments to be made.

La belle indifférence   A lack of affective expression, concern, and insight about a physical problem or significant feelings; the person appears to be inappropriately neutral or bland in the setting of a serious illness or major stressor. Powerful, unconscious psychologic conflicts underlie this affect of indifference when it occurs in the setting of a conversion disorder. It also accompanies some brain disorders, such as multiple sclerosis or frontal lobe disorders. For further discussion, see Chapter 3, under Mood.

Personality   The intangible, yet pervasive and unique, phenomenon in each person that determines his or her character and demeanor—that is, an individual's typical behavior patterns, feelings, and identity. Personality governs and encompasses habitual responses to internal and external stimuli, sense of self (ego), and the ability to realize the boundary between self and other. Personality styles vary greatly among individuals, although they remain relatively constant throughout one's lifetime, except when brain damage occurs. Personality may be partially determined prenatally, but it also develops significantly in stages throughout the lifetime, in coordination with concurrent life experiences and maturation of brain, cognition, and sexuality. Early childhood and adolescence are peak periods for the formation and refining of personality and identity. In "healthy" personality development, there are stages during which different and maturing types of defense mechanisms are utilized (see this section). The normal personality is a balanced mixture of obsessive-compulsive, passive-dependent, histrionic, antisocial, aggressive, altruistic, and narcissistic features, which combine in such a way that no one feature is dominant or excluded. *Personality disorders* involve maladaptive patterns of coping and behaving related to an imbalance of these features that comprise personality, and an inadequate sense of self (or identity). In personality disorders, the likelihood of having healthy interpersonal relationships with the appropriate amount of intimacy is markedly reduced. Persons with personality disorders usually have inadequate insight into their own abnormal behaviors and how these behaviors affect other persons. They have difficulty handling their own mixed or conflictual feelings and often make defective judgments because of distortions in their perceptions of external reality. There is, of course, a continuum between healthy personality styles and severe personality disorder, with varying degrees of abnormality of traits and styles between these two extremes.

Projection   An immature defense mechanism in which the person unconsciously attributes to (projects onto) another person his or her own feelings, ideas, or impulses, particularly the undesirable ones. In this way, the undesirable feelings or opinions are separated from oneself and attached (projected) to another person who is then "blamed" or held responsible for these unwanted feelings. This is a primitive way of thinking and coping, and it occurs in personality disorders, including borderline, paranoid, and narcissistic types, and in psychoses.

Reaction formation   A neurotic defense mechanism in which persons behave exactly oppositely from the impulse they really feel. This behavior occurs because the true feeling, either positive or negative, is unacceptable and undesirable. For example, a person dutifully and zealously cares for an elderly parent who had previously been abusive and whom the person subconsciously hates. Another example is the avoidance of and apparent lack of interest in a person who is unconsciously adored. In each case the true feeling is repressed, having been converted into and outwardly manifested as an opposite behavior.

Repression   A neurotic defense mechanism in which the person appears passively to "forget" an affect-laden and undesirable idea or feeling, thus preventing it from reaching conscious awareness. Usually one component, either the affect or the idea, is repressed or buried in unconsciousness, whereas the other component is apparent but incomplete. The incomplete nature of the conscious idea or feeling makes it difficult for the person to be aware of and insightful about a problematic issue. For example, one may not realize why one is feeling sad because the reason is hidden from conscious awareness. Suppression (see below this section) also involves pushing away undesirable thoughts or feelings, but by purposeful rather than unconscious means. Repression differs from denial in that the repressed component can be discovered and then acknowledged, perhaps through psychodynamic psychotherapy; repressing patients do not reject evidence of the repressed material in the manner that a denying person would. Repression should be differentiated from amnestic syndromes that are due to brain lesions or dysfunction (see Chapter 6).

Resistance   The conscious or subconscious efforts of a patient to avoid self-awareness in the setting of another person's efforts to increase insight. Examples include "forgetting" appointments, arriving late for appointments, denying the validity of the therapist's interpretations, "losing" a prescription, and so on.

Splitting   See Chapter 2 for definition.

Sublimation   A mature defense mechanism that reduces the painful or unwanted effects of certain emotions, impulses, or ideas (e.g., anger) by modifying them and channeling them into a practical activity. Sublimation may be involved in hobbies, artwork, music, teaching, homemaking, and athletics if unwanted emotions are being transformed into useful and pleasurable activities. In contrast to displaced feelings, sublimated feelings are acknowledged and redirected to a more acceptable expression, in a harmless and productive way. Playing tennis for the healthy enjoyment of exercise and the outdoors can be sublimation; if the tennis ball is a substitution for the boss's head, then it becomes displacement. In sublimation, the person is consciously aware of feelings and gains some control or mastery over them.

Suppression   A mature defense mechanism in which the person consciously postpones addressing an idea, impulse, or feeling until a later time; for example, "I'll deal with that problem tomorrow." The uncomfortable thing is not ultimately avoided nor is it unconsciously denied or repressed; rather, it is deliberately and temporarily set aside, and then dealt with at another time. Insight is involved in this process.

References

Vallaint, G. E. *Adaptation to Life: How the Best and Brightest Came of Age.* Boston: Little, Brown, 1977.

8 | Case Examples

The following examples are fictional case descriptions, with relevant historical information in the form of a vignette (as opposed to the standard format for a medical history as listed in Chapter 1) to serve as background information to illustrate sample MSEs as they might be written in a medical chart. The Appendix at the end of the book lists an outline of the headings and major topics for each section of an MSE and can be used as a general guide while writing MSEs.

CASE 1. MAJOR DEPRESSION

Vignette

Anna Black, a 43-year-old married woman, presented to the emergency room on her wedding anniversary with suicidal ideation and a plan. She has been thinking about locking herself in the garage with the car engine running to kill herself. Two months ago, her husband of 20 years told her he was having an affair and wanted a divorce. He moved out of the house and has not been sending her money for household expenses. Their children are away at college and Anna is alone. She has few friends because she had devoted herself to her husband's needs, and now feels helpless and unsupported. For two months she has had insomnia, decreased appetite, a 12-pound weight loss, anergy, decreased libido, low self-esteem, reduced concentration, decreased motivation, and suicidal ideation. She repeatedly mulls over how she has been a bad wife, that the divorce is all her fault, that she is not pretty enough, and so on. She feels she deserves to be denigrated.

There is no prior psychiatric history, drug or alcohol abuse, or active medical problem. Her only medications are aspirin for headaches and over-the-counter sleeping pills.

Mental Status Examination

Appearance, Attitude, Activity Appears stated age, is slightly unkempt, clothes are wrinkled, and not wearing makeup. Is moderately psychomotor retarded, sits slumped in a chair. Eye contact is limited; eyes are downcast. Often tearful and occasionally sobs. Is generally cooperative with the interview.

Mood and Affect Mood is severely depressed and hopeless. Blunted affect, with reduced range. Affect not reactive.

Speech and Language   Speech fluent and grammatical. Decreased spontaneity of speech, with prolonged latency and pauses. Occasional word-finding difficulty. Speaks in a monotone with little prosodic variation.

Thought Content and Process and Perception   Has active suicidal ideation, says "Life is not worth living anymore," but denies homicidal ideation. Content focused on low self-esteem issues and anger at husband. Has guilty ruminations. Denies suspiciousness, delusions, illusions, or hallucinations. No thought disorder.

Cognition   Oriented times three. Attention deficit, with digit span forward = 6, backward = 3. Concentration decreased, four errors on serial sevens. Mild short-term memory deficit, with two out of three objects recalled after five minutes. Mini-Mental State score = 23/30 (mildly impaired). At times gives up easily with cognitive questions; says "I don't know."

Insight and Judgment   Insight impaired by depressive symptoms; views world unrealistically negatively. Judgment is impaired, as evidenced by her suicidality.

CASE 2. PRIMARY DEGENERATIVE DEMENTIA OF THE ALZHEIMER'S TYPE

Vignette

Ms. Sanders, a 72-year-old widow, presents to the geriatric outpatient clinic accompanied by her 45-year-old daughter, with whom she has been living for the past two years. Ms. Sanders has been increasingly forgetful, to the extent that she cannot remember family birthdays, when her husband died, or how many grandchildren she has. She awakens at night and wanders around the house, often confused as to where she is and believing that it is time to get dressed. She misplaces her clothing and then accuses others of stealing from her. Because she believes certain neighbors are breaking into the house to burglarize it, she hides her jewelry and then cannot find it. There is no sign of forced entry, and there are extra locks bolting the doors. Trying to explain that misplacing the items is the more likely explanation for their disappearance has not helped, as she avidly adheres to the theft idea. She is often irritable, a change from previous years. Her personality has also become more rigid and stubborn, and she has hit her daughter during clothing changes. As she has become less able to cook or dress herself, her daughter must perform these tasks for her. Although she denies hearing things that are not there, she claims to have seen strangers taking food out of her refrigerator.

She has never abused drugs or alcohol, and has no prior history of psychiatric disorder. She retired from elementary school teaching 12 years ago. As a result of a motor vehicle accident 15 years ago, she suffered a concussion. She takes medications for hypertension and angina. There is no family history of dementia.

Mental Status Examination

Appearance, Attitude, and Activity Patient appears older than stated age, is unkempt, and smells of urine. Blouse is buttoned asymmetrically. Has an action tremor. Is intermittently agitated and restless, wanting to leave the room. Is only partially cooperative with the interview, and is irritable and occasionally hostile. Acts defensively when cognitive questions are asked. At times seems to be looking at and attending to unseen persons in the room. Tearful once, but incongruent to topic. Daughter answers many of the questions.

Mood and Affect Mood is irritable and aggressive. Affect is labile, rapidly changing from calm to irritable, at one point inexplicably dysphoric. Affect often inappropriate to content.

Speech and Language Speech fluent and grammatical, with prominent word-finding difficulties. Paraphasias common, both semantic and literal. Confrontational naming is impaired, especially for parts of objects.

Thought Content and Process and Perception Not actively suicidal or homicidal. Thought content focused on finishing the interview and on people stealing from her. Persecutory delusions and visual hallucinations present. Thoughts at times are tangential, but no loosening of associations or blocking.

Cognition Is not oriented to date or place, but recognizes self and daughter. Perseverates saying "1929, 1929, 1929 . . ." Severe memory deficits, both short and long term. Attention span decreased, with digit span forward = 4, backward = 3; cannot recite months of year backwards correctly. Does not know U.S. presidents ("Roosevelt"). Named only four items from a grocery store in one minute. Visuoconstructional deficits, unable to draw a clockface or to copy cube. Interprets similarities concretely. Mini-Mental State score = 10/30 (very impaired); Mattis score = 78/144 (very impaired). Is apraxic for buttoning sweater.

Insight and Judgment Insight very impaired due to diffuse cognitive deficits and psychotic symptoms. Is not aware of her illness or the effects of her behavior on daughter. Judgment is impaired owing to dementia and its associated disinhibited behavior.

CASE 3. DELIRIUM

Vignette

Sophie Koszarsky, a 56-year-old diabetic woman, was brought to the emergency room by ambulance, unaccompanied by family or friends, because of chest pain. A chronic smoker, her arterial blood gases revealed hypoxia, an EKG showed inferior wall myocardial infarction pattern, and her lab work was consistent with diabetic ketoacidosis. She denied alcohol abuse. She was combative, punched the doctor, and needed to be restrained.

In her hospital room, she was yelling out "Charlie, Charlie, help me, help me," "They're torturing me," "Don't take my brain." Throughout the day, these periods of agitation alternated with calmer periods and with naps. At times she looked and pointed into the air, picked at her sheets, and talked at the closet door. She reported to the nurses that dogs were at the window (eighth floor), trying to break in. Her sleep was disrupted at night. She was frightened.

Mental Status Examination

Appearance, Attitude, Activity   Disheveled, wearing a hospital gown, lying in bed with intravenous lines and with arms restrained. Has cigarette stains on fingers. Edentulous. Is hypervigilant, her eyes darting around rapidly. Picks at herself and has mild intention tremor. Is minimally cooperative with interview and at times is hostile.

Mood and Affect   Mood is anxious and angry. Affect is labile. Affect ranges from apparent sadness when crying, to irritability, although incongruent to topic.

Speech and Language   At times incoherent and unintelligible. Occasional sentences are grammatical, but not well articulated. Lapses into Polish. Confrontational naming and writing are impaired. Semantic paraphasias present. Comprehension impaired, but repetition intact.

Thought Content and Process and Perception   Content centered on her fears, including being tortured by hospital staff. Has visual hallucinations and possibly also visual illusions; has tactile hallucinations; questionable auditory hallucinations, also. Has persecutory delusions. Not overtly suicidal or homicidal.

Cognition   Disoriented to time, place, and person. Does not recognize family members, thinks it is 1958 and that she is in a restaurant. Severe attentional deficits, can barely attend to the examiner's questions. Difficulty registering information, short-term memory severely impaired, long-term memory impaired for recent and remote events. Thinking is concrete. Visuoconstructional ability impaired, cannot copy cube. Mini-Mental State score = 6/30 (severely impaired). Trailmaking Test Part A = 349 seconds with many errors; incapable of executing Part B.

Insight and Judgment   Both insight and judgment are grossly inadequate because of the delirium and are not even testable at this time.

CASE 4. ALCOHOL ABUSE AND DEPENDENCE

Vignette

Willard Kelly is brought to clinic by his family because "he drinks too much and we are fed up with it." Willard is a 49-year-old ex-steelworker, has been married for 31 years, and has six children. He has abused his family both emotionally and physically throughout his marriage. When intoxicated, he gets irritable and aggressive, occasionally hitting the children or his wife. She has never brought legal charges against him because she has no other source of income and is financially dependent on him. At the encouragement of their grown-up children she began attending Al Anon meetings and learned how she "enabled" her husband to continue his alcohol abuse. Now she wants him to quit drinking or she will divorce him. Recently, he has been accusing her of "cheating on him," although she denies this adamantly.

Mr. Kelly began drinking at 15 years of age with his father, who also worked in the steel mills. He enjoyed the taste of alcohol as well as the way it made him feel. With the burden of supporting six children, he appreciated the sense of escape he felt when drinking. He drinks a fifth of whiskey and a six-pack of beer every weekday and even more beer on the weekends. He begins drinking when he awakens in the morning or else he feels shaky. He has never had a prolonged sober period and has never attended a rehabilitation program or Alcoholics Anonymous. He has lost his license twice because of DWI and driving to endanger. He has had blackouts and one episode of DTs.

His medical history includes a bleeding duodenal ulcer and a subdural hematoma. His father, two uncles, and three brothers all have alcohol problems. His grandmother committed suicide. He does not take any medications, prescribed or illicit.

Mental Status Examination

Appearance, Attitude, Activity   Mr. Kelly looks older than his stated age, with multiple wrinkles and telangiectasia on his face. He is casually dressed in work clothes. Sclerae are mildly icteric. He is tremulous and has an intention tremor. While ostensibly cooperative, he brags and tries to minimize the need for assessment. He has hostile moments. He is fidgety while sitting in a chair. Whenever his wife makes a comment, he glares at her.

Mood and Affect   States that he feels "just fine." Affect is euthymic but mildly anxious and irritable. Range of affect is full, including anger and inappropriate laughter.

Speech and Language   Speech is spontaneous, loud at times, loquacious, and somewhat pressured. It is grammatical and mostly fluent except for occasional mild difficulty initiating words. No paraphasias. Confrontational naming, repetition, and comprehension are intact.

Thought Content and Process and Perception   Content centered on how there is nothing wrong with him; he "just has a few drinks with the boys after work." Doesn't know why his wife made him come to the evaluation. Denies visual, auditory, or olfactory hallucinations. No suicidal or homicidal ideation. No loosening of associations or racing thoughts. Slightly tangential.

Cognition   Oriented times three. Attention intact. Registers 5/5 objects, but recalls only 4/5 after five minutes (got 5th with semantic cuing). Long-term memory mildly impaired. Visuoconstructional ability intact except some impairment with more difficult figures (e.g., Rey–Osterrieth). Mild tremor noted on drawings. Difficulty with proverbs and similarities; tendency to be concrete. Mini-Mental State score = 24/30 (borderline normal).

Insight and Judgment   Very poor insight regarding alcohol abuse. Uses much denial and externalization as defenses. Has difficulty being empathic toward others' feelings and needs. Judgment is also impaired; has driven while intoxicated and continued to drink excessively despite injuring family. Even with threat of losing wife, still has difficulty realizing the extent of his drinking and its consequences. Gastrointestinal effects of alcohol abuse have not motivated him toward abstinence.

CASE 5. ORGANIC PERSONALITY DISORDER, FRONTAL LOBE (AGGRESSIVE) TYPE

Vignette

Jeb Milner was driving home after working late at the office when his car was struck by a truck driving out of control. Not wearing a seatbelt, he hit his head against the dashboard and lost consciousness. X-rays revealed a depressed fracture of the left frontal bone, and CT scan showed cerebral contusion with hemorrhage in the left frontal lobe. A year later, at age 33, he now appears in clinic for evaluation of irritability, decreased concentration, inability to remember his appointments, and temper outbursts. His sales as a stockbroker have greatly decreased because of poor organizational skills and losing his temper with customers. He denies insomnia, euphoria, racing thoughts, or changes in energy level.

Sarah Milner, his wife and mother of their two children, works as an attorney and has had to take on all household responsibilities since Jeb's injury. She is frustrated by his inability to plan or to focus his attention on family needs, and by his decreasing income. They have had more severe and frequent marital strife that twice escalated into Jeb's striking her. He is less sensitive about her needs and does not seem to "get the main point" when they talk. She believes he underwent a personality change after the head injury and is not the man she married. He was previously hard-working, conscientious, polite, and sensitive. He has been uncharacteristically sexually aggressive with her, and she is frightened of him. He loses his temper for minor reasons and has alienated many of their friends. He even has started drinking heavily. When she suggests getting marriage counseling, he fears she will divorce him; he said he might as well drive his car into a concrete bridge abutment.

Jeb has no prior history of psychiatric illness, takes no medications regularly, and is otherwise medically healthy.

Mental Status Examination

Appearance, Attitude, Activity Tall, muscular, slightly balding young man who appears stated age. Neatly dressed in blue jeans and a Dartmouth sweatshirt. At first reluctant to talk, but then cooperative. At one point arose abruptly from his chair and waved his hands in the air, looking frustrated. Threw a pen across the room.

Mood and Affect Mood is dysphoric overall and irritable on occasion. Affect labile, with rapid escalations to anger. Affect full range.

Speech and Language Speech is largely grammatical and fluent, with occasional, slight difficulty initiating words and phrases. Speech is spontaneous with normal prosody; at times somewhat pressured. No paraphasias. Naming, repetition, and comprehension intact.

Thought Content and Process and Perception Not actively suicidal or homicidal; some passive suicidal ideation without current plan. Thoughts centered on fears that he will lose his job and his family. Denies feelings of persecution, suspiciousness, hallucinations, and delusions. No ideas of reference, flight of ideas, or looseness of associations. Some depressive ruminations.

Cognition Oriented to place and person, not know day of month. Attention intact with digit span forward = 7 and backward = 5; serial sevens without errors. Trailmaking Test Part A = 35 seconds, Part B = 170 seconds. Impairment in shifting mental sets on Symbol Digit test. Short-term memory intact with 3/3 words and 5/5 shapes post five minutes. Difficulty generating words beginning with *b* (10 in one minute). Retrograde amnesia for several days preceding and anterograde for events occurring several weeks after the car accident. Knew past five U.S. presidents and recalled his best man and wedding date. Could not abstract proverbs and did not identify similarities between apple and banana or truck and car. Perseverates on Go–No go tapping test. Impaired on Stroop test. Calculates simple additions and rote multiplications well, slight difficulty with more complex calculations. Mini-Mental State score = 28/30.

Insight and Judgment   Poor insight related to difficulty with executive functions (abstract thinking, switching mental sets) and irritability. Poor judgment related to emotional disinhibition, temper outbursts, and impulsivity.

CASE 6. OBSESSIVE-COMPULSIVE DISORDER

Vignette

Betty Scott is a 24-year-old who recently delivered a healthy baby boy, Jason. Jason resulted from an unplanned pregnancy. Before he was born, Betty diligently prepared his room, scrubbing the walls and floors clean. Actually, Betty was perfectionistic about all of her work and had a particular system for performing most chores. When leaving the house, she would check the door several times to see if it were locked. When washing the dishes, she would hold each dish facing the left and then turn it exactly four times during rinsing. Any interruption would "require" her to restart at the beginning of these procedures. She had to resign from her job as a department store clerk because she was too inefficient and spent too much time packaging purchases.

She presented at dermatology clinic because her hands were red, dry, and raw. Since her baby was born, she has been frightened of germs and scrubs her hands repeatedly so as to not infect the baby. She cannot control this urge and is preoccupied with germs. Dermatology referred her to psychiatric clinic.

Betty has insomnia and nightmares about her baby dying; she claims not to be a good enough mother. She feels anxious and tired most of the day. Whenever she fears her baby's death, she washes her hands again. In fact, Betty spends most of her day scrubbing her hands and accomplishes little else. Her husband thinks she has "gone crazy"; if he touches the baby, she wants to wash Jason to avoid contamination. Her husband can get her to admit that her fears are excessive, yet she is overcome by an irresistible urge to scrub repeatedly. She washes Jason only with a particular brand of babywipes, always beginning from the left side because the heart is on that side.

Betty grew up in a strict, highly religious family where sexual topics were repressed. On her honeymoon, Betty was shocked by intercourse and found it repulsive. She has "never touched" drugs or alcohol and denies any past or family psychiatric history. There is no family history of tics or chorea. She is medically healthy.

Mental Status Examination

Appearance, Attitude, Activity Thin, petite young adult woman who looks more like a teenager, with long blonde hair and some acne. Is neatly dressed in casual clothing; blue jeans are pressed with creases. Slightly tremulous, lips quiver, and seems tentative in her interactions. She is cooperative and makes good eye contact. There is mild psychomotor agitation; fidgets in chair, with baby on her lap. Her hands are chapped. No tics, mannerisms, compulsions, or choreiform movements.

Mood and Affect Mood is dysphoric and anxious. Affect has reduced range; does not smile or laugh during interview.

Speech and Language Speech is fluent and grammatical, at times with decreased prosody. Spontaneous, but sometimes pressured and difficult to interrupt. Comprehension, repetition, and naming intact.

Thought Content and Process and Perception No suicidal or homicidal ideation. Obsessed and preoccupied with germs and fears about death or contamination of baby, but not of delusional proportions. Tangential and circumstantial. Has magical thinking about wiping baby certain way. Denies auditory hallucinations commanding her to wash; no visual or tactile hallucinations, or illusions. No ideas of reference, blocking, or looseness of associations.

Cognition Oriented times three. Distractible, but when focused, attention is intact. Serial sevens = 5/5; digit span forward = 7, backward = 5. Short-term memory intact; 3/3 objects and 5/5 shapes post five minutes. Long-term memory intact; knew past five U.S. Presidents. Abstractions intact for similarities but proverbs only partly abstract. Mini-Mental State score = 29/30.

Insight and Judgment Obsessional thinking and compulsive urges interfere significantly with insight into abnormality of thinking and symptoms. Also, magical thinking decreases insight. Judgment impaired as evidenced by rituals and chapped hands.

CASE 7. PARANOID SCHIZOPHRENIA WITH ACUTE EXACERBATION

Vignette

Harry Payton, a 29-year-old single man, was brought to the emergency room by the police on an emergency involuntary commitment. Harry had been threatening to his roommate in a group home for the mentally ill. Harry had lived in the group home since his discharge from the state hospital seven months ago. The home's supervisor reports that, at first, Harry was quiet and aloof, but was calm, neat, inoffensive, and tolerant of his roommate. Things worsened about three months ago; complaining of pain in his buttocks, Harry persuaded a physician to discontinue the long-acting fluphenazine decanoate medication and switch to oral perphenazine. It is not clear whether he has been taking the medicine, but for at least two months he has been more haphazard in dress, his thinking has become more disorganized, he has been up much of the night pacing and watching TV, and he sleeps more during the day. There were about half a dozen loud arguments with his roommate about the light being on, too much noise, and allegedly stolen cigarettes. For the last week Harry mutters to himself, limps, and yells "That's bullshit!" at the television. On the day of admission, Harry accused his roommate of stabbing his feet while he slept. He then threatened his roommate with a knife which he had just purchased; he later surrendered the knife without argument when the police arrived. The boarding home personnel are frightened by his violent threats.

Harry was a 23-year-old graduate student studying engineering when he was hospitalized for the first time because he threatened his neighbors. At that time, he had "heard" his neighbors ridiculing and talking about punishing him. He believed that they tampered with his stereo equipment when he was out and had devised a method of reading his thoughts. Although these hallucinations and persecutory beliefs were suppressed by antipsychotic medication, he dropped out of school and has never worked. He has had four or five subsequent hospitalizations lasting from one to four weeks each; each followed his discontinuation of his medication. Harry is in good physical health. Both his paternal grandmother and father's brother died in a state hospital, but other family members have been healthy and successful. He experimented occasionally with marijuana and LSD in college, but has completely avoided drugs or alcohol "for religious reasons" since his first hospitalization. EEGs and brain scans have been normal.

Mental Status Examination

Appearance, Attitude, Activity Appears stated age, unshaven, hair un-combed, mildly malodorous, clothes clean but rumpled, and shirt tails out. Sits with arms crossed; avoids eye contact and repeatedly scans room; startled by noises several times, but otherwise shows no psychomotor agitation. Patient was noted to speak out loud several times to nobody in particular while in the waiting room.

Mood and Affect Patient is worried and mildly hostile. Affect is blunted and restricted to uncomfortable/angry/suspicious range, but mobile within this range. Affect is appropriate to the content of thought.

Speech and Language   Speech is spontaneous and fluent, but monotonous and sometimes scarcely audible. Perseveratively repeats "I didn't mean that" and "But he crippled me."

Thought Content and Process and Perception   Thoughts are tangential and circumstantial, with occasional loosening of associations. No blocking is noted. Preoccupied with the "danger" he has faced: He feels that his roommate has been injecting poison into his arches while he sleeps, that someone has been stealing thoughts from his mind. Believes that the interviewer can read his thoughts, and expresses hope that he will not be punished for the insults that he "didn't mean." Believes the TV broadcasts special messages for him. Denies hearing voices during interview, but says that passing motorists have been threatening and insulting him. No visual, tactile, or olfactory hallucinations. Denies suicidal or homicidal ideation.

Cognition   Fully oriented, digit span forward = 6, backward = 4; Concentration is decreased, with two errors on serial sevens. Remembers 3/3 objects at five minutes and presidents back to Kennedy. Accurate with similarities, but unable to abstract any but the simplest proverbs.

Insight and Judgment   Insight poor; delusionally believes he is in danger, denies need for hospitalization or that he has ever been mentally ill; blames hospitalizations on the malevolence of others. Poor judgment, as demonstrated by his threats and noncompliance with medication.

CASE 8. BIPOLAR DISORDER, MANIC

Vignette

Sherri Johnson, a 32-year-old substitute teacher, was brought to the emergency room by her husband after several days of manic symptoms of increasing severity. She had severe gastroenteritis during the previous week, and had discontinued all of her medications, including lithium, at that time. Over the preceding three days, she has slept no more than one to two hours per night. Her husband describes her talking more rapidly, being more irritable, and frequently taking drinks from the liquor cabinet. Earlier in the day she had a loud argument with a neighbor; subsequently, she repeatedly voiced concerns that her neighbors were "spying" on her when she danced around her bedroom naked. She has been flirtatious with male teachers at school and joking inappropriately. She believes that a Las Vegas talent scout will soon be auditioning her for her dance routine.

Sherri's father had several hospitalizations for bipolar disorder before his suicide at age 51. Sherri has been generally successful at school, in her work and marriage, and in raising her children. However, she has had three episodes of depression, each of which responded to treatment with tricyclic antidepressants. After one of these depressive episodes, she had experienced a manic episode with grandiose delusions, requiring hospitalization. She has no drug or alcohol abuse and is physically healthy.

Mental Status Examination

Appearance, Attitude, and Activity This is a young, slightly obese white female, dressed casually but wearing makeup. She frequently walks about the room, and gesticulates vigorously while speaking. She is partially cooperative with the exam, but says that she came in only because her husband insisted and that she "feels wonderful and doesn't need a doctor." At times, she appears to dance.

Mood and Affect She is cheerful and describes her mood as "great." She is very expressive of her cheerful mood, but affect is mildly labile, with several angry comments and irritability when interrupted by the examiner. Affect is appropriate to thought content but inappropriate to her situation.

Speech and Language Speech is loud and pressured. Fluent and grammatical. Normal prosody.

Thought Content and Process and Perception Tangentiality bordering on flight of ideas. Preoccupied with her anger toward her neighbors, that they might interfere with the talent scout. Suspicious about her neighbors. Has grandiose delusions, feeling that others are jealous of her looks and dancing ability, and that she will soon have an entertainment job in Las Vegas. Denies hallucinations, suicidal ideation, or thoughts of harming others.

Cognition Alert and fully oriented. She is intermittently distractible and performs poorly on serial sevens, and refuses to answer long-term memory questions, but recalls 3/3 objects at five minutes. Normal performance on similarities and proverbs. Refuses to draw a clockface.

Insight and Judgment Acknowledges that "I need to get back on my lithium," but minimizes mood and thinking disturbances and does not readily see the connection between stopping her medications and her current condition. Believes that talent scout will be coming soon, even though this is extremely unrealistic. Enjoys her euphoria and does not see a problem.

| Appendix

General Outline of Written MSE Report

Appearance, Attitude, Activity
  Describe appearance:
    Body habitus
    Prominent physical characteristics
    Grooming and attire
    Level of consciousness
    Apparent age
    Position and posture
    Eye contact
    Facial expressions
  Describe attitude:
    Degree and type of cooperativeness
    Resistance
  Describe activity:
    Voluntary movements and their intensity
    Involuntary movements
    Automatic movements
    Tics, mannerisms, compulsions
Mood and Affect
  Describe predominant mood:
    Six clusters (euthymic, apathetic, angry, dysphoric, apprehensive,
      euphoric)
  Describe affect:
    Type
    Intensity
    Range
    Mobility
    Reactivity
    Congruency
Speech and Language
  Evaluate for aphasias and other primary disorders of language
  Evaluate for secondary language symptoms
  Assess for:
    Fluency of speech
    Repetition

Comprehension
Naming
Reading and writing
Prosody
Quality of speech

Thought Content, Thought Process, and Perception

Describe thought processes:
Degree of connectedness (loose associations, tangentiality, etc.)
Presence of peculiarities (clang associations, blocking, neologisms, etc.)
Describe thought content:
Predominant topic or issues
Delusions
Preoccupations/ruminations/obsessions
Suicidal/homicidal ideation
Phobias
Describe perceptual abnormalities:
Illusions
Hallucinations
Depersonalization, déjà vu, etc.

Cognition

Assess for:
Orientation
Attention and concentration
Calculations
Short-term memory
Long-term memory
Visuospatial and constructional ability
Abstraction and conceptualization

Insight and Judgment

Describe insight:
Effect of psychiatric symptoms or defense mechanisms on capacity for
insight
Insight about any psychosocial or medical problems and current
psychiatric illness
Describe judgment:
Reasoning regarding current important issues
Ideas about decisions or actions to be taken, including about current
illness
Evidence from past judgments as clues to current thinking

Index

Note: Numbers set in **boldface** type indicate page numbers where terms are defined.